DATE DUE

MAR 24 1995	MAY - 6 1997
APR - 5 1995	OCT - 7 1997
APR 20 1995	FEB 23 1998
NOV - 6 1995	DEC 1 5 1998
DEC - 6 1995	MAR 15 1999
Dec 20/95	Nov 22
JAN 9/96	APR 1 8 1999
JAN 17 1996 Jan 31/96	FEB 1 6 2000
Feb 14/96	MAR - 1 2000
Feb 28/96	APR - 4 2000
	APR 1 2 2000
MAR 1 4 1996	OCT 1 0 2000
APR 1 1 1996	Morgan-Nicole
AUG 0 1 1996	due May 11/01
FEB 1 1 1997	Fraser Valley Reg
MAR - 3 1997	due Dec 1/02
APR - 9 1997	

Borderline Personality Disorder

A
Multidimensional Approach

Borderline Personality Disorder

A
Multidimensional Approach

JOEL PARIS, M.D.
Associate Professor of Psychiatry
Sir Mortimer B. Davis–Jewish General Hospital
Department of Psychiatry, McGill University
Montreal, Quebec, Canada

American
Psychiatric
Press, Inc.

Washington, DC   London, England

Note: The authors have worked to ensure that all information in this book concerning drug dosages, schedules, and routes of administration is accurate as of the time of publication and consistent with standards set by the U.S. Food and Drug Administration and the general medical community. As medical research and practice advance, however, therapeutic standards may change. For this reason and because human and mechanical errors sometimes occur, we recommend that readers follow the advice of a physician who is directly involved in their care or the care of a member of their family.

Books published by the American Psychiatric Press, Inc., represent the views and opinions of the individual authors and do not necessarily represent the policies and opinions of the Press or the American Psychiatric Association.

Copyright © 1994 American Psychiatric Press, Inc.
ALL RIGHTS RESERVED
Manufactured in the United States of America on acid-free paper
97 96 95 94   4 3 2 1
First Edition

American Psychiatric Press, Inc.
1400 K Street, N.W., Washington, DC   20005

Library of Congress Cataloging-in-Publication Data
Paris, Joel, 1940–
    Borderline personality disorder : a multidimensional approach /
Joel Paris. — 1st ed.
      p.   cm.
    Includes bibliographical references and index.
    ISBN 0-88048-655-4
    1. Borderline personality disorder—Etiology. 2. Borderline personality disorder—Risk factors. 3. Borderline personality disorder—Treatment.
I. Title.
    [DNLM: 1. Borderline Personality Disorder—etiology. 2. Borderline Personality Disorder—therapy. WM 190 P232b 1994]
RC569.3.B67P37 1994
616.85′852—dc20
DNLM/DLC   93-48728
for Library of Congress   CIP

British Library Cataloguing in Publication Data
A CIP record is available from the British Library.

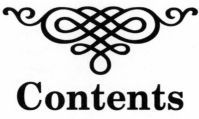

Contents

Acknowledgments ix

Introduction xi

1   Definition and Boundaries 1

2   Personality Traits and Personality Disorders 11

3   Biological Risk Factors 27

4   Psychological Risk Factors 43

5   Social Risk Factors 69

6   A Multidimensional Theory of Borderline
Personality Disorder 87

7   Outcome 99

8   Treatment Options 109

9   Clinical Management 133

10   Research Directions 155

References 163

Index 193

*To
John Gunderson*

Acknowledgments

Special thanks are due to the American Psychiatric Press, Inc., who supported the idea of this book. In particular, I have received practical help from the Editor-in-Chief, Carol Nadelson, M.D., and from the Editorial Director, Claire Reinburg.

The time to write the text was provided through generous support from the Sir Mortimer B. Davis–Jewish General Hospital, Montreal, and its Psychiatrist-in-Chief, Philip Beck, M.D., as well as from the Department of Psychiatry of McGill University and its Chairman, Gilbert Pinard, M.D.

Every author is dependent on the help of friends and colleagues who are willing to read earlier drafts and suggest improvements. I had the benefit of three critical and helpful readers: Rosalind Paris, John Sigal, and Hallie Zweig-Frank, all of whom suggested many useful improvements in the text.

I would like to acknowledge a special debt to Hallie Zweig-Frank, who first encouraged me to undertake research on borderline personality disorder, with whom I have collaborated on many studies, and who helped me to clarify most of the ideas in this book.

I learned most of what I know about scientific methodology from the members of the research group at the Department of Psychiatry of the Sir Mortimer B. Davis–Jewish General Hospital. Laurence Kirmayer convinced me that I could actually write a book on borderline personality disorder. Jim Robbins taught me to understand multivariate statistics. Our librarian, Ruth Stillman, helped me find crucial references.

Laura Rose helped me transfer an earlier draft of the text to the computer. Zeev Rosberger answered all my questions about word processing, which allowed me to revise this book.

I am particularly grateful to the members of the personality disorders research community who have stimulated my ideas about the understanding and investigation of borderline personality disorder. I would like to make special mention of John Gunderson, who pioneered the empirical investigation of borderline personality disorder and who has continued to be a leader in research on the personality disorders. Although there are many other colleagues who have profoundly influenced me, I would like to give particular acknowledgment to Allen Frances, Marsha Linehan, Paul Links, John Livesley, Thomas McGlashan, Theodore Millon, Larry Siever, Kenneth Silk, Michael Stone, and Mary Zanarini. Finally, the ideas in this book are derived from the contributions of some of the innovators in psychiatric theory. One name that requires special mention is that of Sir Michael Rutter.

I would like to express my gratitude to my family for their support during the writing of this book. In particular, I am indebted to my wife, who believed at an early stage that I could make a successful career as a psychiatrist.

Earlier versions of some of the ideas in this book have been published in a series of articles that have appeared in the *Canadian Journal of Psychiatry* (Paris 1992, 1993b; Paris and Zweig-Frank 1992), as well as in the *Journal of Personality Disorders* (Paris 1993a).

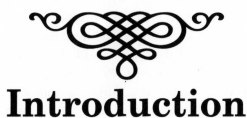

Introduction

The Purpose of This Book

There is an enormous literature on borderline personality disorder (BPD). However, little of what has been written is firmly grounded in scientific research, and the etiology of the disorder is essentially unknown. Many well-known theoretical formulations remain at best plausible hypotheses. Moreover, borderline patients are notoriously difficult to treat. Much of what has been suggested thus far for their management has proved impractical in the majority of cases.

This volume is addressed to readers who are skeptical of facile explanations and who are not easily satisfied with expert recommendations. The book has two overall goals:

1. To build a comprehensive theory of etiology that takes into account biological, psychological, and social factors.
2. To suggest treatment guidelines that are consistent with this theory and that are based on the findings of clinical trials.

To this end, we will review in 10 chapters what is known about the etiology, outcome, and treatment of BPD. For most of the book, research findings will be given greater weight than clinical experience. This focus on empirical evidence is deliberate. When we attempt to explain problems in individual patients, we do not require proof, and it is sufficient to obtain clinical confirmation of a hypothesis. But to draw conclusions that can be generalized to groups of patients, we must study large numbers of cases and apply scientific methods. No theory that attempts to explain BPD can be based on unsystematic clinical observations. This is why we cannot rely on the conclusions of clinicians, however prestigious, whose databases consist of the intensive therapy of a few selected cases. As Aronson (1989) has noted, "From a methodological perspective, almost the entire treatment literature overgeneralizes from small patient samples, uses inconsistent diagnostic criteria, and relies heavily on anecdotal, uncontrolled, unsystematic, personal experience" (p. 524). Because so many of the books published on BPD fit this description, it is not surprising that their recommendations have proven less than useful for clinical practice.

A Multidimensional Approach

Borderline personality disorder is a complex construct. Its etiology is most likely multifactorial, and there is no single definitive therapy. Therefore, a comprehensive approach to the disorder has to consider multiple dimensions. Unidimensional psychiatric theories fail to account for the etiological pathways that lead to psychopathology. Nor do such theories provide useful guidelines to the complexities of clinical management. Therefore, this book, in contrast to many others on the subject, will examine BPD in a multidimensional framework.

Unidimensional theories are reductionistic but attractive. They offer easily comprehended explanations and may imply a clear course of treatment. Psychiatry is not unique in being attracted to simple paradigms. In medicine, explanations of disease often attempt to approximate linear models such as the germ theory of infection and the one-gene–one-enzyme model of hereditary illness. In reality, few diseases, including infectious and hereditary conditions, can be well understood using such simple paradigms. Most medical illnesses are better accounted for by multidimensional models. An example would be myocardial infarction, in which many risk factors, including heredity, diet, smoking, life stress, and personality, all contribute to a pathological outcome.

A multidimensional framework has in fact been applied to many medical illnesses (Weiner 1977). The theory suggests that illness develops from the interaction of multiple risk factors. Many people with these predispositions never develop illness. Among those who do become ill, there is individual variation as to which risk factor is most important.

This framework is highly relevant to psychiatry. The major mental disorders, such as schizophrenia and depression, derive from multiple risk factors and rarely respond to one modality of treatment. Moreover, prospective studies of children have shown that children do not develop psychopathology as adults unless they are exposed to several risk factors (Rutter and Rutter 1993).

The personality disorders require a multidimensional approach. As this book will attempt to show, these complex disorders are shaped by biological vulnerability, brought on by psychological experiences, and influenced by social conditions.

The Biopsychosocial Model

The multidimensional approach to psychiatric disorders is essentially identical to a biopsychosocial model (Engel 1980). This model implies that psychopathology develops from multiple risk factors, including biological vulnerability, psychological experiences, and social influences. Each risk factor may be necessary, but none is sufficient to lead to a specific disorder. In addition to these risk factors, there may be protective factors against psychopathology, which in turn can be biological, psychological, or social (Rutter and Rutter 1993). All of these multiple factors interact in a complex pathway, such that their assessment requires multivariate studies to consider simultaneously the effects of many variables on the same outcome.

In spite of its obvious advantages, the biopsychosocial approach has not been applied systematically to the study of mental disorders. Clinical psychiatrists tend to be primarily either biological or psychosocial in their orientation to the etiology and treatment of psychopathology. Researchers also tend to be trained in particular methods, and most studies have measured single risk factors in univariate designs.

Clinical and research perspectives that take the biopsychosocial model seriously also require wide theoretical knowledge and a tolerance for cognitive dissonance. Although psychiatric training aims to be eclectic, many psychiatrists still seem to belong to "schools." This theoretical fragmentation is a barrier to progress in psychiatry. It reflects an early stage of scientific development, in which investigators rely on authority rather than on paradigms that lead to testable hypotheses (Kuhn 1970).

Neo-Kraepelinian Theory

The dominant paradigm of North American psychiatry is based on neo-Kraepelinian theory (Klerman 1986). This model, although not strictly based on the ideas of Emil Kraepelin, follows his empirical and phenomenological approach to the mental disorders. Neo-Kraepelinians consider psychiatric diagnosis to be categorical, and they begin by establishing precise boundaries for each diagnostic entity. They then search for biological markers that are associated with a specific vulnerability to that disorder. Treatment tends to be biologically oriented and specifically targeted at constitutional vulnerabilities. The neo-Kraepelinian paradigm contrasts with psychodynamic theory, which tends to emphasize the role of specific psychological experiences in shaping psychopathology.

The construct of biological vulnerability can explain why the same psychological experiences lead to entirely different disorders in different individuals (Cloninger et al. 1990). Neo-Kraepelinian theory is a predisposition-stress model in which biology determines the specificity of mental disorders and psychological and social stressors are precipitants that exert a nonspecific effect (Cloninger et al. 1990). If it could be shown that there are specific psychological or social factors for a psychiatric diagnosis, the model would require modification. One of the questions to be examined in this book is whether the neo-Kraepelinian model is appropriate for personality disorders in general or for BPD in particular.

In conceptualizing the etiology of BPD, we need to distinguish between necessary and sufficient conditions. There seem to be a number of necessary conditions for developing BPD. It will be argued in this book that biological factors are necessary for psychopathology to take the particular form seen in borderline patients, but that the presence of this biological vulnerability does not by itself lead to BPD. The evidence that psychological factors are required for vulnerable individuals to develop borderline psychopathology will be reviewed. Social factors may also either increase or decrease the possibility of developing the disorder. Only a combination of these risks would be a sufficient condition for the development of BPD. This multidimensional model will be shown to shed light not only on the etiology but on the natural history of BPD and its response to treatment.

The Argument of the Ten Chapters

Chapter 1 addresses the problem of defining the boundaries of BPD. One difficulty is the misleading term "borderline," which is a bad name for this disorder but which is nonetheless familiar to clinicians. There have also been problems with the construct of BPD, and it remains fuzzy around the edges. There is a troublingly high comorbidity with other disorders, both on Axis I and Axis II. There are those who do not think that BPD is a valid diagnostic category at all. It will be shown that although BPD does not, in fact, meet rigorous criteria for diagnostic validity, its position in this regard is no worse than that of most of the disorders in the *Diagnostic and Statistical Manual of Mental Disorders* (DSM). The diagnosis has a clinically important degree of predictive validity in that borderline patients have a characteristic course of illness and response to treatment. The problems with the borderline construct are better understood, however, if we apply both dimensional and categorical approaches to diagnosis. To do so requires an understanding of personality dimensions, which is the subject of the next chapter.

Chapter 2 concerns the relationship between personality traits and personality disorders and provides a theoretical scaffolding that will be used throughout the rest of the book. Personality traits are universal. Because traits vary continuously in their intensity, they can be measured as dimensions. The major theories of personality dimensions are reviewed in terms of their relevance to the understanding of personality disorders. The basic dimensions of personality may eventually be described more precisely, but based on analyses of the symptoms seen in borderline patients, the core dimensions of BPD seem to be *impulsivity* and *affective instability*. The relationship of personality dimensions to BPD can help unravel some of the problems in its definition. The core dimensions will also be shown later in the book to help explain the role of the risk factors for BPD, as well as the outcome and treatment of the disorder.

In the next three chapters, the biological, psychological, and social risk factors for BPD are examined. Chapter 3 reviews the question of whether there are biological vulnerabilities for BPD. There is, in fact, little evidence for a specific genetic pattern or for any specific biological markers in BPD. In general, it is the traits that underlie personality disorders that reflect genetic factors, and evidence for the heritability of personality dimensions will be reviewed. The core dimensions of impulsivity and affective instability could reflect the biological risk factors for BPD. However, these traits most likely are necessary but not sufficient conditions for the development of BPD.

Chapter 4 examines the psychological risk factors for BPD. Several of these factors, including trauma, loss, and abnormal parenting, have been studied empirically. Because sexual and physical abuse during childhood have been shown to be particularly frequent in borderline patients, it has been proposed that childhood trauma has a specific relationship to BPD. Evidence from research carried out both by the author and by others is brought to bear to demonstrate that the evidence does not support a linear relationship between traumatic risk factors and BPD. Most likely all of the psychological risk factors that have been studied play some role in the etiology of BPD, but none of them have a very specific link to borderline psychopathology.

Chapter 5 addresses the subject of social risk factors in BPD. The social environment has not been the subject of empirical research in borderline patients, and the evidence for its role is indirect. Epidemiological findings are presented which suggest that the prevalence of BPD is increasing and that social factors could be implicated in this change.

There are also theoretical reasons to expect that the core dimensions of BPD are sensitive to social context. It will be hypothesized that the mechanism by which social factors increase or decrease the risk for borderline pathology involves the construct of social disintegration.

Chapter 6 attempts to integrate the biological, psychological, and social risk factors in a multidimensional model of the etiology of BPD. The general theory is presented that personality disorders are maladaptive amplifications of personality traits. The biological factors in personality disorders are reflected in these traits. The underlying dimensions of personality are a limiting factor for what type of personality disorder could develop in any individual. Environmental risk factors, including psychological experiences as well as disturbances in the wider social network, determine whether traits are amplified to dysfunctional levels. Applying this theory to BPD, there would be an interaction between biological factors (traits of impulsivity and affective instability) and psychological risk factors (trauma, loss, or abnormal parenting), as well as with social risk factors (social disintegration). BPD would be a final common pathway in which a number of environmental risk factors act together to elicit pathology in vulnerable individuals.

Chapter 7 examines the long-term outcome of BPD and reviews a number of studies that have followed borderline patients well into middle age. It will be shown that BPD is a chronic disorder with high morbidity and mortality but that its symptoms decline with age. A likely mechanism for improvement involves maturational changes in the core dimensions of impulsivity and affective instability. The evaluation of treatment methods for BPD must be considered in the context of this naturalistic recovery.

Chapter 8 reviews the treatment options for borderline patients. The primary point of reference will be the findings of clinical trials. A series of possible therapeutic strategies in BPD will be critically reviewed. Psychopharmacological interventions, although based on well-designed studies, seem thus far to be of marginal utility. Hospitalization of borderline patients is also of doubtful value. In evaluating the various forms of psychotherapy that have been recommended for patients with BPD, there have been too few clinical trials to reach any solid conclusions, and even the best research is limited by the samples of patients studied and the lack of long-term follow-up. It is also not known whether the positive effects of psychotherapy in BPD are related to specific techniques or to nonspecific effects that are common to many methods. It is argued in this chapter that psychodynamic psychotherapy is best reserved for a small subpopulation of borderline patients and that recommendations of intensive therapy as the treatment of choice for borderline patients have been seriously misleading for therapists. It is also suggested that most borderline patients do better with treatment that is supportive and intermittent. There seems to be no therapy of choice, and treatment planning must take into account the heterogeneity of BPD.

In Chapter 9 these conclusions are applied to the development of guidelines for the clinical management of borderline patients. A longitudinal approach is taken, starting from evaluation and ending with posttermination follow-up. The principles of management are 1) to predict treatability, 2) to control symptoms, 3) to establish structure, 4) to encourage the development of competence, and 5) to follow patients intermittently after discharge. In the absence of firm research findings, these principles are illustrated by clinical vignettes drawn from the author's clinical experience with a wide variety of borderline patients.

Chapter 10 summarizes the conclusions of the earlier chapters and offers suggestions for future directions of research. There are many unanswered questions about BPD. This volume offers a number of theoretical proposals about the etiology and treatment of this disorder. These hypotheses will have to be confirmed or disconfirmed by empirical research. The aim of this book is to promote inquiry, not certainty.

1

Definition and Boundaries

A Psychiatric Misnomer

Borderline personality disorder (BPD) is a psychiatric misnomer. The term developed out of the theory that there is a realm of psychopathology that lies on a border between neurosis and psychosis (Stern 1938). Because this concept is now something of a historical curiosity, the continued use of the term "borderline" has led to enormous confusion.

To be fair, BPD is far from the only mental disorder to be badly named. Schizophrenia is an obvious example in which the name of a disorder obscures its essential clinical features. The histories of the terms "borderline personality disorder" and "schizophrenia" parallel each other in that in each case the original construct on which the name was based was jettisoned but the label was retained. The use of the term schizophrenia causes misunderstanding outside psychiatry, and psychiatrists themselves would have to re-read Bleuler (1911/1950) to know what he meant by a "split mind." But we still speak of schizophrenia because the term has a strong clinical tradition. Although we are stuck with a misnomer, we can define it with fairly precise criteria. We can thank (or blame) Adolf Stern (1938) for introducing the term "borderline" into psychiatry. His clinical description included phenomena that are still recognizable characteristics of the borderline patient: narcissism, "psychic bleeding," inordinate hypersensitivity, psychic rigidity, negative therapeutic reactions, feelings of inferiority, masochism, "wound licking," somatic anxiety, projection, and difficulties in reality testing.

Nevertheless, for the next 35 years the concept of a "borderline patient" remained exclusive to the analytic literature. The diagnosis did not appear in either DSM-I (American Psychiatric Association 1952) or DSM-II (American Psychiatric Association 1968). The psychopathology described by Stern continued to be treated under other diagnostic names, such as "hysteria" or "pseudo-neurotic schizophrenia" (Hoch et al. 1962). The construct of BPD lacked both a clear theoretical foundation and a clinical tradition.

In the 1960s, one of the author's most esteemed teachers advised rather strongly against applying this diagnosis to patients, commenting archly, "After all, nobody knows what it means." At that time there were no diagnostic criteria for borderline personality, and much of the literature on patients with this diagnosis described metapsychological phenomena that were not open to observation.

But the problem with avoiding this diagnosis is that even if the disorder is poorly defined, there are still borderline patients. Whatever we call them, these patients are characterized by impulsivity, affective instability, and unstable relationships, and this pathology forms a recognizable clinical syndrome. The diagnosis of BPD also has enormous implications for outcome. Borderline pathology follows a highly chronic course and is notoriously resistant to treatment. One would happily use a term other than "borderline," but the entity would still exist. As Linehan (1993) points out, changing the name will not change the clinical problem.

Operational Criteria for the Borderline Diagnosis

A turning point for the definition of BPD came in the 1970s. Gunderson and Singer (1975) were the first to develop a truly operational definition of BPD. Their description was based on those characteristic clinical features that had been noted in the literature and that could be reliably observed and scored. Gunderson's group at McLean Hospital later showed that BPD could be distinguished from other major mental disorders (Gunderson and Kolb 1978) as well as from other personality disorders (Zanarini et al. 1989a, 1990b). Once borderline personality could be reliably diagnosed, research on borderline patients grew exponentially, and BPD became the most investigated of the personality disorders.

By 1980 the construct was strong enough to earn inclusion in DSM-III (American Psychiatric Association 1980). When the disorder was first accepted into the American psychiatric classification in 1980, there was discussion of what name to use. Spitzer et al. (1979) proposed the reasonable term "unstable personality disorder" and polled American psychiatrists to test its acceptability. As it turned out, a majority of the respondents were still most comfortable and familiar with "borderline personality disorder." In a narrow vote by the DSM-III committee (T. Millon, personal communication, 1991), "borderline personality" was retained. In part the decision reflected clinical usage, but it was also a concession to psychoanalysis, which was already feeling sufficiently bruised by the elimination of the concept of "neurosis."

However, the retention of the term "borderline" has had a long-term negative impact on the acceptance of the construct. The psychoanalytic concept of a continuum between all forms of psychopathology, from the mildest to the most severe, runs counter to the tenets of neo-Kraepelinian psychiatry. When disorders are defined by their phenomenology, there is no border on which to be borderline. In addition, the term "borderline" has divided North American from European psychiatrists, for whom it lacks a clinical tradition. In a book on personality disorders, the British researcher Peter Tyrer (1988) noted that BPD leaves non–North Americans with a feeling of "bemusement." This is not to say that borderline patients do not exist in Europe. Kroll et al. (1982) showed that these individuals form a sizable percentage of admissions in Britain, but that they were labeled differently there. Simonsen (1993) has also shown that borderline psychopathology is common in several European countries. But outside the United States and Canada, BPD has been the subject of major research only in Scandinavia.

Recently BPD has been accepted into the *International Classification of Diseases,* 10th Revision (ICD-10; World Health Organization 1992). It is classified there as a subcategory of "emotionally unstable personality disorder," a more phenomenological term that resembles the "unstable personality" that was nearly accepted into DSM-III. The construct of emotionally unstable personality disorder also comes closer to capturing two of the crucial dimensions of BPD: impulsivity and affective instability.

The definition of BPD in DSM-IV (American Psychiatric Association 1994) requires the presence of five criteria from a list that includes the original eight from DSM-III-R (American Psychiatric Association 1987): frantic efforts to avoid abandonment, unstable relationships, identity disturbance, impulsiveness, suicidal threats, affective instability, emptiness or boredom, and inappropriate anger. In addition, a ninth criterion—"transient, stress-related paranoid ideation or severe dissociative symptoms"—was added (American Psychiatric Association 1994, p. 654). The original DSM-III definition had been criticized on several grounds, including that it was written by a committee, that it combines several theoretical perspectives, and that it allows too many ways to reach the same diagnosis (Clarkin et al. 1983). These objections can be partly met by empirical studies that aim to increase the reliability and validity of each criterion and that make the criteria more specific to the diagnosis (Gunderson et al. 1991).

One of the best ways of achieving reliability in diagnosis is through semistructured interviews. There are a number of these instruments, which are used to diagnose all of the Axis II disorders, although these instruments are not highly reliable with each other (Perry 1992). The Diagnostic Interview for Borderlines (DIB; Gunderson and Kolb 1978) was specifically designed for BPD and has been widely used to make research diagnoses. In its revised version, the DIB-R (Zanarini et al. 1989a), the responses on 136 questions are scored on four scales: affect, cognition, impulsivity, and interpersonal relationships, and BPD is defined by a cut-off point (8 out of 10) on the total score.

There is little doubt that BPD is a useful clinical construct. The term is sufficiently meaningful that therapists who work with personality disorders can often make the diagnosis within minutes of meeting the patient. The practical importance of identifying BPD patients is that the construct predicts important aspects of clinical course and re-sponse to treatment. However, there remain important problems for the diagnostic validity of BPD.

The Validity of Borderline Personality Disorder

One problem regarding the validity of BPD is that the DSM criteria sets for the personality disorders prior to DSM-IV were based more on clini-cal tradition than on systematic research. An attempt was made by the DSM-IV Axis II subcommittee to establish the discriminant validity of all existing and proposed criteria (Gunderson et al. 1991). There is a side effect to these improvements, since even the smallest change in criteria can cause major effects in the diagnosis of personality disorders (Blashfield et al. 1992), leading to disruptive effects on clinical research (Zimmerman et al. 1991).

Unlike the major Axis I diagnoses, Axis II diagnoses have no single required criterion. Choosing any five out of eight or nine possible cri-teria, as one does for BPD, has been called a "Chinese menu" approach (Frances and Widiger 1986). When diagnosing personality disorders, clinicians do so prototypically (Livesley 1986; Morey and Ochoa 1989)—that is, they look for features that resemble the most typical case. A definition of BPD based on a prototype would give stronger weight to its most typical features rather than simply list and count them. However, in the absence of a strong empirical basis for such a prototypical definition, the present criteria have remained unweighted.

The definition of BPD may also depend excessively on affective dysphoria, leading to a spurious overlap with mood disorders (Kroll 1988). The clinical prototype of BPD that most clinicians actually use (Morey and Ochoa 1989) would give a stronger weighting to impulsive actions and unstable relationships. The presence of transient stress-related paranoid ideation or severe dissociative symptoms was added in DSM-IV because these phenomena have been shown to usefully dis-criminate BPD from other personality disorders (Zanarini et al. 1989a, 1990a).

The DSM-IV criteria for BPD are a compromise; they are not based on a theory. In the next chapter the suggestion is made that if we could define which personality traits or dimensions are abnormal in BPD, we would have a better grounding for our definition. Evidence will be presented later in this book for the hypothesis that impulsivity and affective instability are core dimensions that underlie BPD. If these traits could be shown to be crucial factors in borderline personality, they would be made pathognomonic in the criteria.

Another problem for the validity of BPD is whether it is a syndrome or a disorder. A syndrome is the co-occurrence of symptoms that can be produced by many different psychopathological processes. An example is congestive heart failure, which has a defined clinical course but arises from many etiological sources. Disorders, on the other hand, have a specific etiology.

In two classical papers, E. Robins and Guze (1970) and Feighner et al. (1972) proposed a multiphase method for defining valid psychiatric disorders. These approaches were neo-Kraepelinian manifestos that influenced an entire generation of psychiatrists (Blashfield 1984) and established the conceptual basis for DSM-III. The criteria that should be met to determine if a diagnostic entity is valid fall into five phases: 1) clinical description, 2) laboratory studies, 3) delimitation from other disorders, 4) follow-up studies, and 5) family studies.

The clinical description of BPD has been fairly well established. Although subgroups of borderline patients can be identified, many studies have shown that the overall syndrome includes symptoms that co-occur frequently and form a recognizable pattern (Zanarini et al. 1989a).

As will be reviewed in Chapter 3, there are no laboratory findings that are specific to BPD, and there are reasons to doubt that BPD has a discrete biological nature.

The issue of delimitation from other disorders is thorny. The problem of delimiting BPD from Axis I disorders will be discussed later under the topic of comorbidity. Many studies (Nurnberg et al. 1991; Oldham et al. 1992; Pfohl et al. 1986) have also shown major overlap between BPD and other Axis II disorders. However, this problem could lie more in the structure of DSM diagnostic rules than in the nature of BPD. For example, if we were to prohibit multiple Axis II diagnoses and only use that category in which the largest number of criteria were satisfied, the overlap would diminish. Such hierarchical rules, when applied to Axis I diagnoses such as schizophrenia and bipolar mood disorder, increase diagnostic specificity. At present we just do not know enough to justify doing the same for Axis II (Gunderson et al. 1991). But in practice, as Blashfield and Herkov (1993) have shown, most clinicians are not interested in any other personality diagnosis once they recognize BPD.

Follow-up studies, as we will see in Chapter 7, have demonstrated that BPD has a reasonably specific course that differentiates it from many other disorders.

As we will see in Chapter 3, family studies suggest that it is not BPD, but impulsive disorders as a group that run in families.

Therefore, BPD does not at present fulfill either the Feighner or the Robins and Guze criteria for diagnostic validity. Nevertheless, it would be premature to demote BPD to a syndrome. In fact, the vast majority of the DSM-III-R disorders, including major depression (Akiskal 1991), fail to meet these criteria. We should not apply a higher standard to BPD than to other major diagnoses. We have a gold standard for diagnostic validity, but the real world is made of copper.

Comorbidity: Explanation or Artifact?

Comorbidity refers to the presence of two mental disorders in the same patient. It might better be called "co-occurrence," because there is no reason in theory why patients should have only one psychiatric diagnosis. However, when comorbidity is present we must ask whether the features of one disorder could account for those of another. The frequent comorbidity of BPD has led some psychiatrists to oppose the use of the diagnosis. There are neo-Kraepelinian psychiatrists who propose that the phenomena we call "borderline" can be accounted for by comorbid diagnoses on Axis I. There are also psychodynamically oriented psychiatrists who believe that BPD could be understood as a chronic posttraumatic stress disorder (PTSD).

Akiskal (1991) has been a prominent spokesman for the first group. He views Axis II disorders in general as milder forms of Axis I pathology and has suggested that the phenomenology of BPD can best be explained as a variant of affective disorders (Akiskal et al. 1985). This view has a number of theoretical implications (Kroll 1988). While Axis I has become dominated conceptually by the neo-Kraepelinian approach to psychopathology, Axis II has been more or less a residual psychodynamic enclave (Gunderson and Pollack 1985). If the personality disorders are nothing but variants of Axis I disorders, then our theoretical models of these conditions might become more strongly biological.

The hypothesis that BPD can be reduced to a variant of mood disorder was rejected in a comprehensive review by Gunderson and Phillips (1991). It would be worthwhile to recapitulate their arguments. Although there is comorbidity between BPD and major depression or dysthymia, such comorbidity with depression also exists for all the other personality disorders. BPD is infrequent among depressed patients, which suggests that the relationship between BPD and depression is nonspecific. There is an important difference between the phenomenology of depression in borderline and nonborderline patients, with BPD patients describing more emptiness and loneliness and having a mood that is more environmentally responsive. Family history studies (to be reviewed in Chapters 2 and 3) do not strongly support a link between mood disorder and borderline personality. As will be discussed in Chapter 8, borderline patients do not respond to antidepressants in the same way as do patients with mood disorders. There are no clear-cut biological markers for BPD, and those markers shared with depression are only present when the patient shows major depression or dysthymia. Finally, there is stronger evidence for environmental loading in BPD than in mood disorders. Gunderson and Phillips concluded that BPD and depression co-occur but are not otherwise related.

A peculiarity of the concept of comorbidity is that it is often assumed that when Axis I and Axis II disorders coexist, the Axis I disorder has etiological primacy. Certainly, depression exaggerates and distorts personality characteristics (Frances and Widiger 1986). However, it is equally important to consider how personality disorders influence mood. Depression is, of course, not simply a function of biological vulnerability, but is elicited by environmental triggers. In BPD, pathological interpersonal relations are the most common environmental events that produce depression.

Recognizing comorbidity has the advantage that individual characteristics of patients are given consideration. But too much emphasis on comorbidity obscures identification of the constructs that organize and give meaning to complex patterns of psychopathology. Borderline patients can have multiple Axis I comorbid diagnoses, and clinical experience even suggests that the more Axis I diagnoses there are in a chart, the more one should consider whether the patient has BPD! It is not clinically meaningful to make multiple diagnoses of anxiety disorders, mood disorders, and substance abuse in the same patient when a single organizing construct, borderline personality disorder, makes sense of all the symptoms and is a better predictor of treatment response.

The other question is whether there is an overlap between BPD and PTSD. Herman and van der Kolk (1987) have suggested that patients with BPD who have strong histories of childhood trauma could be reclassified as having chronic PTSD. Kroll (1993) has gone so far as to relabel this clinical group as "PTSD/borderline" patients. As will be discussed in Chapter 4, this formulation is highly premature, given our lack of knowledge about the etiology of BPD. It should be noted that PTSD is one of the few Axis I diagnoses in which a specific cause is built into its definition. Therefore, to redefine BPD as a PTSD would be to assume that we know the etiology of BPD, when in fact we do not.

In summary, the evidence reviewed in this chapter provides support for the clinical usefulness of borderline personality disorder as a diagnostic category. However, its validity as a disorder still leaves a great deal to be desired. The construct should be retained because of its clinical utility, but it needs to be refined.

The most serious question is whether BPD is one thing or many things. This is a general problem for the personality disorders, which can be understood either as constituting discrete categories or as consisting of multiple dimensions. In the next chapter, the dimensional approach to diagnosis will be discussed in the context of the relationship of personality traits to personality disorders.

2

Personality Traits and Personality Disorders

Personality traits are consistent patterns of behavior, emotion, and cognition that characterize individuals. These traits are ubiquitous in individuals and demonstrate variability within populations. A distinction should be made between *temperament*, which describes characteristics present from birth, and *traits*, which are amalgams of temperament and experience (Rutter 1987). But personality traits are significantly influenced by temperamental variations. As will be discussed in Chapter 3, traits have been shown to be under strong genetic influence and therefore reflect, in part, the biological factors in personality.

Personality disorders are diagnosed only when traits significantly interfere with functioning. These disorders can therefore be considered as exaggerations or distortions of underlying traits such that the behaviors deriving from these traits come to be applied rigidly and maladaptively. Thus, there are preexisting traits behind every personality disorder.

The intensity of personality traits can be measured by scores on psychological instruments, in the context of which these traits are termed personality dimensions.

11

Personality Disorders as Categories and Dimensions

Personality disorders are categorical constructs, and a single diagnostic decision will place patients either inside or outside their boundaries. Categories have the advantage of being easier to conceptualize, and they are familiar ways of ordering phenomena. On the other hand, reducing diagnosis to a simple yes-no decision leads to a loss of information about the unique characteristics of patients. This is of particular significance for BPD, in which there may be significant heterogeneity among those individuals meeting the diagnostic criteria for the disorder (Clarkin et al. 1992).

The phenomenology of any personality disorder can also be understood as a reflection of the interaction of a number of separately measurable dimensions. These dimensions offer an alternative method of classification for the personality disorders. A dimensional system avoids the difficulties implicit in using categories, but it does so at the price of making diagnosis more complex. In such a system, patients receive not a label but a set of scores. Personality disorders are defined by cut-off points on dimensions beyond which dysfunction would be expected, much as we define hypertension as a blood pressure value beyond a normative range.

Personality dimensions measure the intensity of personality traits, and there is a wide range of scores that could be entirely compatible with normality. The assumption of dimensional classification is that there is a continuous relationship between personality traits and disorders, such that disorders only represent the extremes of a continuum. There is some empirical evidence for this view (Livesley et al. 1992). It follows that each personality disorder could have a specific relationship to preexisting traits, which would then act as limiting factors for the type of personality disorder that could develop. If we could identify those traits that are unusually intense in patients with personality disorders, it would help to improve our definitions of these diagnostic entities.

Dimensional Theories of Personality

Personality dimensions are usually measured through self-report questionaires. Because some personality characteristics are not apparent to those who have them, one can also score observations from semi-structured interviews. In addition, there are ways of measuring traits through their behavioral consequences. For example, personality dimensions are reflected in defense styles, which are consistent patterns of responding to environmental challenge. Defense styles have been shown to show specific differences in more severe personality disorders such as BPD (Bond 1990; Bond et al. 1994; Perry 1991).

Most dimensional measures of personality are derived from questionnaires describing wide ranges of behaviors and attitudes. Factor analysis defines the dimensions by describing the common characteristics of large numbers of intercorrelated items, such that dimensions are ideally imagined as orthogonal (i.e., uncorrelated). In models that are based on preexisting personality theories, a small number of factors tend to be extracted that measure the broadest aspects of personality. When a purely descriptive and atheoretical approach is taken, it often produces a larger number of dimensions.

Academic psychology has a long tradition of dimensional approaches to personality. There have been many different models, the most important of which are summarized in Table 2–1. Although these systems may seem at first to be contradictory and confusing, there is a reasonable degree of consensus about the broadest factors.

One of the most influential models has been the schema of Hans Eysenck (1990, 1991). Eysenck described three broad factors in personality: extraversion, neuroticism, and psychoticism. Extraversion is defined by sociability, liveliness, and impulsiveness. Eysenck hypothesized that individuals who score low on this dimension (i.e., introverts) have high baseline levels of arousal that lead them to limit interpersonal stimulation, whereas those who score high (i.e., extraverts) have low baseline levels of arousal and tend to seek out interpersonal stimulation. This construct and the theory behind it resemble a dimension that Zuckerman (1979) termed "sensation seeking." Eysenck further hypothesized that extraverts would show differences in evoked potentials re-

Table 2–1.　Dimensional theories of personality

Author(s)	Dimensions	Related to temperament	Heritability	Linked to disorders
Eysenck	Neuroticism Extraversion Psychoticism	Yes	Yes	No
Costa and McCrae	Neuroticism Extraversion Openness to experience Agreeableness Conscientiousness	Yes	Yes	No
Buss and Plomin	Emotionality Activity level Sociability	Yes	Yes	No
Millon	Active-passive Subject-object Pleasure-pain	Probably	?	Yes
Cloninger	Novelty seeking Harm avoidance Reward dependence	Yes	Yes	Yes
Leary and Wiggins	Affiliation Dominance	Probably	?	No
Tellegen	Positive emotionality Negative emotionality Constraint	Yes	Yes	No
Siever	Impulsivity-aggression Affective instability Anxiety-inhibition Cognitive-perceptual	Yes	Probably	Yes

flecting the activity of the reticular activating system, as well as increased dopaminergic activity. There is some evidence for both of these hypotheses (Stelmack 1991).

Neuroticism includes traits such as moodiness and anxiety and is a measure of emotional stability. Eysenck suggested that this trait reflects limbic system activity. The interaction of the dimensions of extraversion-intraversion and neuroticism has been shown by Eysenck to lead potentially to a re-creation of Galen's four temperaments: the melancholic, choleric, phlegmatic, and sanguine personalities.

The third dimension, psychoticism, is something of a misnomer, because it focuses on traits such as insensitivity to others and may in fact relate more to psychopathy than psychosis.

Recently, the most influential dimensional theory of personality has been the concept of the five personality factors developed by Costa and McCrae (1988). The "big five" dimensions, as measured by an instrument called the NEO-PI, are neuroticism, extraversion, openness to experience, agreeableness, and conscientiousness. The first two dimensions are essentially the same as Eysenck's. Openness to experience relates to imaginativeness. Agreeableness is an interpersonal construct that relates to emotional warmth. Conscientiousness relates to behavioral control and is the inverse of impulsivity.

These models describe the broadest dimensions of personality. As will be discussed later, these dimensions delineate adult personality characteristics that are largely attributable to variations in temperament. A dimensional model that is explicitly based on aspects of temperament that can be observed in early childhood has been developed by Buss and Plomin (1984). In their model these authors proposed that emotionality, activity level, and sociability (EAS) are the key elements of personality. (Impulsivity was included in an earlier version of the schema but was later considered a more complex construct lying at the interface of more basic dimensions.) Sociability is similar to extraversion, and emotionality parallels the construct of neuroticism. Activity level is another major variable in temperamental observations of infants and was included in the schema developed by Chess and Thomas (1984).

A very different biologically based model of personality dimensions has been proposed by Millon (1981). This schema is based on three sets of polarities—active-passive, subject-object, and pleasure-pain—motivational systems that are grounded in evolutionary theory. The 11 permutations of these three factors, when associated with dysfunction, tend to correspond to the Axis II categories. Millon's model therefore allows for the coexistence of dimensional and categorical systems.

A more specific biological model for personality dimensions has been developed by Cloninger (1987). The Tridimensional Personality

Questionnaire (TPQ) is an instrument that measures dimensions of novelty seeking, harm avoidance, and reward dependence. These factors correspond in theory to the actions of three major neurotransmitters (dopamine, serotonin, and norepinephrine, respectively). Novelty seeking is related to extraversion and stimulus seeking. Harm avoidance, the converse of impulsivity, refers to concern with the negative consequences of action. Reward dependence relates to concern about the opinions of other people. Cloninger, like Millon, used the permutations of these dimensions to reconstruct a categorical system.

The problem with the Cloninger schema is that, thus far, the evidence for the relationship of these particular neurotransmitters to behavior is unclear. First, there are not just three neurochemical systems in the brain. Second, there are different receptor systems for each transmitter, each with different behavioral effects. Third, each neurotransmitter may have different actions at different sites in the brain (D. L. Murphy et al. 1990). As recently acknowledged by Cloninger and colleagues (1993), the original system was too simple and has now been revised into a less biologically based seven-dimensional schema that includes both temperament and "character."

Another important system based on the relationship of personality dimensions to neurotransmitter activity has been developed by Larry Siever (Siever and Davis 1991). Because this schema has been tested primarily on patients with personality disorders rather than in normal populations, it will be discussed later in the chapter.

There is evidence that the personality traits identified by psychological inventories do have biological roots. There have been specific tests of the genetic factors in personality dimensions for virtually all of these schema through twin studies. Heritability of about 50% has been demonstrated by this method for the Eysenck model, Costa and McCrae model, the EAS model, and the Cloninger dimensions. There is also strong heritability for several other models to be discussed below (Livesley et al. 1992, 1993; Tellegen et al. 1988; Torgersen et al. 1993). The implications of the heritability of traits will be discussed in greater detail in Chapter 3.

It is also possible to build models of personality that are purely phenomenological. For example, one can define dimensions that describe characteristic patterns in adult interpersonal behavior. The "circumplex" interpersonal theory developed by Leary (1957) was such a model, and it has been revived by Wiggins (1982). Circumplex theory defines two dimensions of interpersonal behavior: affiliation and dominance. Personality traits are therefore characterized by individual attitudes toward closeness and power. The interaction of these factors can be mapped in a series of concentric circles that vary with the strength of the dimensions. The traits that determine affiliation and dominance are stable in a variety of relationships. However, this purely interpersonal model does not describe the cognitive and affective components of personality.

Benjamin (1992) has proposed a more complex interpersonal model with an increased number of dimensions that aim to account for personality disorders as well as for traits. The Structural Analysis of Social Behavior (SASB), a triple circumplex based on intrapsychic theories, describes how behavior reflects internal models of self, other, and introjects.

A number of researchers have taken a less theoretical and more clinically descriptive approach to the dimensions of personality. These systems tend to produce larger number of factors. Tellegen et al. (1988) described 11 dimensions, which can be be reduced to three superfactors: positive emotionality (which parallels extraversion), negative emotionality (which reflects emotional stability), and constraint (which is similar to conscientiousness). Livesley et al. (1989, 1992) have described 18 dimensions derived from factor analyses based on normal populations and on the phenomena seen in patients with personality disorders. Two European schemas, derived from instruments that measure the dimensions of personality pathology (Torgersen et al. 1993; Tyrer 1988), have 16 and 24 dimensions, respectively. These multidimensional schemas may be more useful for researchers than clinicians, because large numbers of factors are usually too complex for practical application.

The main problem with all of the dimensional theories of personality is that they may be more useful in describing normal personality than abnormal personality. In the next section we examine the question of whether dimensional methods can be used to diagnose personality disorders.

The Dimensions of Personality Disorders

Can the present classification of personality disorders be replaced by a dimensional system? From a practical point of view, dimensional diagnosis would work best when the fewest factors are used, such as in the models developed by Eysenck, Costa and McCrae, Buss and Plomin, and Cloninger. The question is whether these broad dimensions can properly account for the complex phenomena seen in personality disorders.

There have been several attempts to convert the Axis II system to dimensions, with the most success having been achieved with the five factors of Costa and McCrae (Costa and Widiger 1994; Soldz et al. 1993; Wiggins and Pincus 1989). In principle it would be possible to replace our present categories with the dimensions described by the NEO-PI. But would five scores do justice to the complexity of personality pathology? One possibility is that five factors are not enough. The overall scores on the NEO-PI can be broken down from five overall factors into 30 "facets." Theorists such as Benjamin (1992) have argued that a larger number of dimensions is required to describe clinical populations. Tyrer (1988) needed 24 dimensions to describe all of the personality disorders.

Livesley (see Livesley et al. 1989), a strong proponent of dimensional diagnosis, has described his work as a method of investigating the "factorial structure" of Axis II. But the problem remains as to whether complex schemas are practical for clinicians.

Another approach to identifying the dimensions of personality disorders is to analyze the symptoms of patients with different personality disorders to determine what common traits can be used to distinguish them from one another. This involves either factor analysis of symptom scores or cluster analysis to describe which patients have symptoms in common. These methods derive their dimensions from the intercorrelations of phenomena measured in clinical populations. For example, in one of these approaches (Torgersen and Alnæs 1989), four dimensions (extraversion-intraversion, neuroticism, controlled-careless, and reality weakness) were derived from cluster analysis of the symptoms of a sample of patients with personality disorder. The permutations of these dimensions were then used to create a categorical system of 16 personality disorders.

As one can readily see, dimensional systems for the diagnosis of the personality disorders can become quite complex. This is probably why, in spite of the possible advantages of a dimensional approach, the categorical system in Axis II has been maintained. After the appearance of the DSM-III, Frances and Widiger (1986) suggested that the problems of the Axis II system could best be solved if it were dimensionalized. But in the end, the DSM-IV retained the personality disorder categories, partly because psychiatrists are trained in a categorical medical system, partly because it is easier in general to communicate about complex phenomena in categorical terms, and partly because it is not clearly established that the dimensional systems in existence can account for Axis II pathology. The more conservative option, to improve the criteria sets for the categorical system, is the basis of the improvements in DSM-IV (Gunderson et al 1991).

The Coexistence of Categories and Dimensions

We can now better answer the question of whether the personality disorders are better classified using categories or dimensions. The whole dispute is reminiscent of controversies over definitions of intelligence in psychology. In that case it has been strongly argued that because intelligence can be divided into separate factors, we should drop the construct of IQ and speak only of "intelligences" (H. Gardner 1977). However, the construct of general intelligence remains valid in view of the fact that these factors are far from orthogonal—that is, there is always a strong intercorrelation between abilities. An intermediate view would be that both sides are right and that there are both general and specific intelligences.

If we apply this analogy to BPD, we see that although there is a factorial structure to BPD, the overall construct reflects the intercorrelation of these factors and could be considered a "superfactor." The whole point of describing patients as having BPD is that impulsivity, affective instability, and relationship problems go together. In none of the cluster-analytic studies of BPD were these dimensions uncorrelated. This is precisely why the overall concept has discriminant validity in relation to other personality disorders. From a clinical point of view the syndromal clustering of the factors is the reason why clinicians continue to find BPD a useful construct.

Those who favor a strictly dimensional approach to the personality disorders include researchers such as Livesley and colleagues (1989), who believe that the present system should be discarded entirely, and Clarkin and Kernberg (1993), who have argued for a dimensional construct called borderline personality organization (BPO), which would put the entire range of personality disorders on a continuum of ego strength versus ego weakness. However, it seems more reasonable to consider that dimensional and categorical definitions provide us with different kinds of information. As Tyrer (1993) has concluded, we need both approaches and should attempt to reconcile them.

The coexistence of categorical and dimensional approaches has some practical implications for research. Whether we are studying etiology or treatment, we could examine data from both points of view. The problems of categorical diagnosis are not unique to Axis II. For example, both depression and anxiety can be seen either as dimensions or as categories in a neo-Kraepelinian system. There are advantages both ways.

In the case of BPD, as we will see in Chapter 3, a dimensional approach seems to be most useful in examining biological substrates. As will be discussed in Chapter 4, a number of important psychological factors in BPD have been identified using a categorical approach. Most of the literature that will be reviewed in Chapters 7 and 8 on the outcome and treatment of BPD is based on categorical diagnosis, but it will also be proposed that the dimensions of BPD are helpful in understanding the course of the disorder and its response to therapy.

The Dimensions of Borderline Personality Disorder

How well can the dimensional approach account for the phenomena of BPD? There have been few studies applying the most important dimensional models of personality to patients with personality disorder. There have been reports using the NEO-PI (Clarkin et al. 1993; Soldz et al. 1993) that BPD subjects are most characterized by an extremely high score on neuroticism, a finding that also confirms the results of an earlier study using the Eysenck Personality Inventory (EPI) (J. C. Perry and Cooper 1985). On the NEO-PI, borderline patients also score low on both agreeableness and conscientiousness, and tend to score high on extraversion (Clarkin et al. 1993; Wiggins and Pincus 1989). Cloninger and colleagues (1993) found that on the TPQ, borderline patients score high in novelty seeking, low in harm avoidance, and low in reward dependence. However, none of these dimensional patterns are entirely specific to BPD, nor do these scores adequately describe all the clinical phenomena of BPD.

Several studies have taken the clinical symptoms of BPD and reduced them to underlying dimensions by factor analysis. Two investigations (Livesley and Schroeder 1991; Hurt et al. 1992) produced similar results. Livesley and Schroeder (1991) found four factors underlying BPD: impulsivity, affective dysphoria, cognitive deficits, and identity diffusion.

Livesley and Schroeder (1991) also examined the relationship between their 18 personality dimensions and a borderline diagnosis. The highest correlations were obtained for affective lability, labile anger, interpersonal lability, and labile self-concept. Lability seems to be quite characteristic of borderline patients and applies to affect, relationships, and identity.

Hurt et al. (1992) found three clusters of BPD symptoms. The first, an identity cluster, comprised symptoms of identity diffusion, feelings of emptiness and boredom, and intolerance of being alone. The second, an affective cluster, comprised symptoms of labile mood, uncontrolled anger, and unstable interpersonal relationships. The third cluster described impulsivity.

In attempting to define the core dimensions of BPD, it is instructive to see which aspects of the borderline construct are seen as prototypical by clinicians. Morey and Ochoa (1989) examined why clinicians diagnose personality disorders even in the absence of the full criteria described in DSM-III. For BPD the most significant symptoms that led to this "overdiagnosis" of BPD were recurrent suicidal gestures and self-damaging impulsivity, with affective instability also reaching significance.

These symptom clusters derived from clinical observation have an important relationship to one of the biologically based dimensional theories of personality discussed earlier in this chapter. Two of the clusters, impulsivity and affective instability, are precisely those that have been proposed by Siever and Davis (1991) as the "core dimensions" of BPD.

From a clinical point of view, impulsivity (i.e., the tendency to act on one's emotions) is a defining feature of BPD. Impulsivity is a dimension of personality that is more specific and narrowly defined than the broader factors described above: straddling several aspects of temperament (Plomin et al. 1990), impulsivity has been described as a facet of neuroticism in the five-factor model (Costa and McCrae 1988) and could also be related inversely to conscientiousness. However, impulsivity could be a clinically relevant personality dimension, having, as will be discussed later, been empirically shown to be associated with biological markers (Coccaro et al. 1989).

Affective instability, which has some relationship to neuroticism, is also a complex dimension. In the borderline patient, clinical observations indicate that mood is highly dependent on environmental reinforcers and is therefore unstable (Gunderson and Phillips 1991).

The other clusters of symptoms seen in BPD, such as identity diffusion and cognitive impairment, are not entirely accounted for by these core dimensions, although it is possible that problems in identity could be in part the consequences of impulsivity and affective instability (Linehan 1993). The cognitive phenomena of BPD, on the other hand, seem to be quite separate and may overlap with other dimensions of personality pathology. However, Zanarini et al. (1990a) have shown that these cognitive symptoms, including psychotic episodes, subdelusional paranoid feelings, pseudo-hallucinations, and severe depersonalization, are all highly discriminating between borderline and nonborderline personality disorders. Reducing BPD to only two major dimensions is therefore an oversimplification, but a useful one. Because the factor-analytic studies of BPD symptoms show that impulsivity and affective instability are the most consistent dimensions that can be derived from the clinical phenomena seen in borderline patients, these dimensions could be the underlying traits that must be present for BPD to develop.

Impulsivity and Affective Instability as the Core Dimensions of Borderline Personality Disorder

The hypothesis that impulsivity and affective instability are the core dimensions of BPD has a basis in psychobiological theory (Siever and Davis 1991). Siever's system attempts to account specifically for the Axis II categories by postulating four dimensions of pathology—impulsivity-aggression, affective instability, anxiety-inhibition, and cognitive-perceptual organization—related to the interactions of neurochemical systems associated with serotonin, norepinephrine, acetylcholine, and dopamine, respectively. Although there has been no specific research on the heritability of these dimensions, similar but more narrowly defined traits have been shown to be heritable by Livesley et al. (1993). The first two dimensions—impulsivity and affective instability—are hypothesized to be abnormal in BPD. In this theory impulsivity results from underactivity of the serotonergic system, which controls behavioral inhibition, and overactivity of the noradrenergic system, which is associated with extraversion and sensation seeking. Affective instability would result from the interaction of a hyperresponsive noradrenergic system and increased cholinergic responsiveness. The combination of impulsivity and affective instability would carry a higher risk than either factor alone, and the theory postulates that borderline pathology could lie at the interface of dysfunction in both these systems.

There are a number of clinical features of BPD that could be accounted for by an interaction between the dimensions of impulsivity and affective instability. A combination of these traits could account for the intense dysphoria and acting out that are most characteristic of BPD. The dimensions could also reinforce each other on a psychological level. Affective lability could lead to impulsivity if the dysphoria cannot be contained and must be acted out to discharge negative emotions when it reaches intolerable levels. Impulsivity could also lead to affective lability, because the results of impulsivity are usually negative, creating more feelings of depression and emptiness.

Evidence from family history studies supports the importance of the core dimensions of impulsivity and affective instability. When the presence of comorbid depression in probands is controlled for, the relatives of borderline patients are most likely to have other Axis II Cluster B diagnoses or substance use disorders (Zanarini 1993a). These findings place BPD with a group of "impulse spectrum disorders." However, in another study (Silverman et al. 1991), the relatives of BPD probands had an excess of either impulsive or affective personality traits, suggesting that both dimensions are important for the disorder.

One puzzling aspect of the phenomenology of impulsive personality disorders is that the clinical phenomenology of impulsivity and affective instability depends in part on gender. Most borderline patients (about 75%) are females (Gunderson 1984). Recurrent self-damaging acts (Fabrega et al. 1991), as well as parasuicides (Weissman 1974), occur mostly in females. Impulsive personality traits in males could result in a different behavioral syndrome, such as antisocial personality disorder (ASPD). ASPD has a sex distribution that is a mirror image of that of BPD, with about 80% males (Reid 1978). Although ASPD patients are not described as having affective instability, the disorder is associated with a significant suicide rate (L. N. Robins 1966). However, the ASPD patient is more likely to express impulsivity in actions that are exploitative of others, whereas the borderline patient is more likely to be a victim. Benjamin (1992) found that she could distinguish these disorders based on whether angry behavior was related to fear of abandonment (in the case of BPD) or the wish to get something (in the case of ASPD). Such differences could be based on gender-linked traits, such as aggressivity, that are independent of personality disorder diagnosis, and could provide one possible explanation of the female predominance in BPD.

What prevents us from securely identifying the crucial dimensions of BPD is our lack of understanding of the nature of the biological factors that underlie personality traits. There are good theoretical reasons for associating traits with biological markers, but thus far there is a lack of hard data. When we understand better the biological basis of both normal and pathological personality development, we will be in a much better position to define the boundaries of BPD.

The theoretical argument of this book is that BPD has a biological basis that can be identified on the trait level. As will be shown in Chapter 3, there is not yet sufficient evidence to fully justify this position. However, as will be argued in later chapters, because psychosocial factors also do not adequately explain the development of this disorder, a biopsychosocial theory would better account for BPD. The rest of the book will therefore draw on the most heuristic and readily available hypothesis, Siever's formulation of the core dimensions of BPD. The nature of these dimensions may ultimately be defined rather differently. However, the outlines of a multidimensional theory of BPD would remain the same.

Risk Factors: The Pathway From Traits to Disorders

What determines whether personality traits become personality disorders? To explain how trait variance leads to dysfunction, we need to consider risk factors. These factors could be biological, in that extremes in the intensity of certain traits could put the individual at risk for a personality disorder. The risk factors could be psychological, in that adverse and traumatic life circumstances could amplify traits and lead to psychopathology. The risk factors could also be social, since traits only become dysfunctional in interaction with the environment. In addition to risk factors for a personality disorder, there may be protective factors against the development of a disorder. Biological protective factors would be traits that buffer the effects of impulsivity and affective instability. Psychological and social protective factors would be positive experiences that buffer the effects of negative ones.

The focus of the next three chapters will be to define those risk factors that could have a specific relationship to the development of BPD. In Chapter 6, a multidimensional theoretical model will be presented in which these factors will be considered together.

3

Biological Risk Factors

Paradigms and Personality Disorders

The question of what causes borderline personality disorder has inspired both passion and ideological conviction. BPD has provided a testing ground for competing psychiatric paradigms, particularly biological and psychodynamic theories (Kroll 1988). The present book proposes that there are a number of interacting biological, psychological, and social risk factors for the development of BPD. Some of these may be necessary conditions, but in most cases only some combination of factors will be sufficient to cause BPD.

In this chapter we will consider the role of biological factors in the etiology of the personality disorders in general and then BPD in particular. The evidence will be shown to be indirect but suggestive. Biological vulnerability seems to be linked to underlying traits rather than overt disorders. Thus far no specific biological risk factors have been identified that could specifically predispose to BPD. However, there are theoretical reasons to expect that future investigations could unearth factors that are at least specific to the core dimensions of the disorder. The reasons for that expectation can best be understood in the context of general theories of psychopathology.

Etiological theories in psychiatry need to account for the specificity of psychopathology, that is, why different individuals develop different disorders. The dominant paradigm in contemporary psychiatry, neo-Kraepelinian theory, postulates specific biological vulnerabilities to account for this specificity (Cloninger 1991). The theory contrasts with psychological theories that invoke specific developmental experiences to account for specific disorders. In the neo-Kraepelinian model, psychological or social factors are seen as nonspecific stressors that precipitate a transition from vulnerability to overt psychopathology.

The neo-Kraepelinian theory therefore predicts that each psychiatric disorder should be validated by the presence of biological markers that reflect a specific vulnerability. Although this paradigm has been widely used for Axis I conditions, its application to the etiology of the personality disorders is more recent. The most specific hypothesis, which has been developed by Siever (see Siever and Davis 1991), proposes that levels of neurotransmitter activity are the biological markers for the Axis II disorders. These variations in the activity of neurotransmitter systems could correspond to individual differences in the intensity of personality traits.

As will be discussed in Chapter 4, most individuals with the psychosocial risk factors for BPD do not develop the disorder. Although some of the most important psychoanalytic theorists of BPD (Kernberg 1984; Stone 1980, 1993a) have proposed theories in which constitutional factors play a major role, others, in their psychodynamic theories of etiology, have assumed some specific relationship between childhood experiences and the development of borderline pathology (Adler 1985; Masterson and Rinsley 1975). The problem with these formulations is that many of the same negative experiences in childhood are highly prevalent in patients who have entirely different disorders and can also be found in individuals with no mental disorder (Anthony and Cohler 1987; Rutter 1989). One advantage of a model of biological vulnerability for BPD is that it can explain these observations. If biological factors are what account for specificity, the disorder cannot develop in their absence.

An important caveat about the application of a neo-Kraepelinian model to the personality disorders is that even if biological factors explain why patients develop BPD and not some other disorder, it would not justify a reductionistic biological explanation for borderline psycho-pathology. Two important points should be kept in mind. First, the genetic shaping of personality traits does not reflect the actions of single genes, one for each possible trait. In fact, the inheritance of personality traits probably corresponds to a polygenetic pattern, similar to that de-scribed for intelligence, for several medical disorders, and for functional psychoses (Gottesman 1991). This means that there is no simple path-way from genes to traits. Second, personality disorders are not that heritable. The study of intelligence offers a useful analogy to explain why this is so. There is good evidence that the heritability of IQ in the general population is about 50% (Scarr and Yee 1980). However, at the extremes of variation, for the disadvantaged and for the brightest, there could be a larger environmental and a weaker genetic contribution (Bouchard et al. 1990). In the same way, if personality disorders repre-sent extreme variations in personality traits, their development may involve less genetic loading and a greater weight of environmental risk factors.

No clear pattern of inheritance for the personality disorders has yet been described. What evidence there is for genetic factors in Axis II disorders, such as antisocial, avoidant, and schizotypal personalities, is in each case associated with criteria that reflect underlying traits (McGuffin and Thapar 1992). In a series of studies of differences in concordance between monozygotic and dizygotic twins for both person-ality categories and dimensions, Torgersen (1980, 1983, 1984; Tor-gersen et al. 1993) found that although the categories lacked a genetic pattern, personality dimensions were strongly heritable. These findings make the most sense if the biological factors in the personality disorders are on the trait level. We shall therefore examine in some detail the research findings on the behavioral genetics of personality.

The Genetics of Personality

The new science of behavioral genetics (Plomin et al. 1990) has pro-duced a large body of research that demonstrates the biological factors in personality traits. However personality dimensions are defined, they are strongly heritable. The most common method for determining the heritability of personality dimensions is by comparing their frequency in monozygotic and dizygotic twins. The results show that for almost any personality trait, monozygotic twins have a much higher concordance. There is a statistical measure, *heritability*, that can be derived from these data. This figure has been around 0.4 to 0.5 for most traits, which means that about half the variance in most personality traits can be attributed to heredity. Heritability figures derived from adoption studies are somewhat lower.

Because personality traits are most likely influenced by the interaction of several genes, differences between monozygotic and dizygotic twins pick up genetic effects for traits that do not run in families, since they only appear when multiple genetic factors are present (Lykken et al. 1992). In addition, it could be that present research methods underestimate the true proportion of personality variance accounted for by genetic influence, because some of the residual variance may involve an interactive effect of genes and environment. As suggested by Scarr and McCartney (1983), children can influence the quality of their own environment by shaping the responses of others to conform to their preexisting traits.

The most striking study ever performed on the heritability of personality was reported by Tellegen et al. (1988). The design combined the advantages of twin and adoption studies by examining monozygotic and dizygotic twins who had been reared together or apart. The correlations between scores on the 11 dimensions measured were just as high regardless of whether the identical twins were raised in the same family or separated at birth. Fraternal twins, like nontwin siblings, had surprisingly little correlation between their personality traits. Tellegen's model-fitting analyses showed that the heritability of most personality traits is close to 50%. There was one interesting exception: there was only a moderate (30%) heritability for a measure of social closeness or intimacy. As Plomin et al. (1990) pointed out, this trait may not be accounted for by heritable superfactors such as extraversion or neuroticism, and could be open to more environmental influence.

Another striking finding of twin studies is that the environmental contribution to personality is mostly "unshared" (i.e., not related to living in the same family). For example, the Tellegen et al. study showed that siblings are about as similar or dissimilar in personality traits regardless of whether they are brought up separately in adoptive homes or in the same family. That environmental effects are unshared could mean that siblings receive different treatment from their parents, that differences in their traits lead them to perceive their environment differently, or that there are important influences on personality that are derived from experiences outside the family. Extrafamilial influences on personality development have been underestimated in the past (Rutter 1989). Whatever the explanation, these findings point to the need for modifications in strictly environmental theories of human development, particularly those that assume a crucial role for family experiences. The effects of childhood development on adult personality can be better understood in interaction with temperamental factors. Personality is more influenced by genetic variations in temperament than had been previously believed.

Necessary and Sufficient Conditions for Borderline Personality Disorder

The findings from behavioral genetics that personality traits are inherited suggest a theoretical explanation for why, even in the presence of negative environmental risk factors, some individuals will develop BPD and some will not. The presence of trait vulnerability would be a necessary but not a sufficient condition for BPD. These traits, which are under genetic influence, would constitute the biological vulnerability for the disorder. However, in the absence of psychological and social risk factors, these biological risk factors alone need not lead to psychopathology. Only a combination of multiple risk factors would be a sufficient condition for the development of BPD.

Let us assume, for example, that BPD-prone individuals inherit traits that make them more impulsive and more affectively labile. Given a normal environment, these traits might only lead to personality characteristics such as activity, liveliness, and emotionality. With a negative environment, such traits could be amplified to the point at which they become dysfunctional. But without some preexisting level of impulsivity and affective lability, even the worst environment would not produce BPD.

Let us also imagine an individual who has a different set of personality traits, characterized by introversion and low emotionality. Again, in the presence of a normal environment, such traits need not produce psychopathology. However, with a negative environment, the traits become amplified to a point at which a personality disorder could develop. However, the resulting disorder would not fall in the impulsive cluster, but in either the A (odd) or the C (anxious) cluster. Biological vulnerability would therefore be a necessary but not a sufficient condition for personality disorder and would determine not whether the individual develops such a disorder but what specific form it takes. The interactions between personality traits and psychological environment will be discussed again in Chapter 6.

Adaptive and Maladaptive Personality Traits

An important implication of this argument is that personality traits by themselves are not pathological; they can be adaptive or maladaptive under different circumstances (Beck and Freeman 1990). Personality traits are clusters of characteristic behaviors. Like anatomical and physiological traits, behaviors are influenced by genes, can be expected to show variance within populations, and are shaped by natural selection. At the extremes of variability, behaviors can be maladaptive and may even interfere with reproductive capacity, at which point the responsible genes would be eliminated from the population pool. However, a wide variety of traits exist within populations, probably because behaviors that are socially maladaptive in one setting can be adaptive in another.

This crucial point is worth examining in some detail. Of course not all features of an organism are adaptive, because they may be incidental accompaniments of other adaptive traits (Gould and Lewontin 1979). However, the assumption of adaptationism for features that otherwise seem nonadaptive is a highly heuristic concept. Genotypic variation cannot be interpreted in terms of a single idealized environment; its interpretation requires an interactional perspective that considers a wide range of possible environments (Dupré 1987; Lewontin 1974). An example from medicine is that diabetes mellitus may reflect a physiological variability that is adaptive in an environment where starvation is endemic, but leads to pathology in an environment where food is plentiful (MacDonald 1988).

Impulsivity as a trait could be adaptive or maladaptive under different circumstances. The maladaptive aspects of impulsivity are fairly obvious in BPD and its related disorders in the impulsive cluster of Axis II. Yet, impulsive behaviors can also be adaptive. A rapid behavioral response is necessary under a number of circumstances. It has been suggested, for example, that there are war heroes who present as having antisocial personality disorder (ASPD) in the context of peacetime society (Yochelson and Samenow 1976). It could be that impulsive traits, associated with lower autonomic thresholds for anxiety (Mednick and Moffit 1985), are useful in conditions of danger, when thoughtful or considered responses are in fact nonadaptive.

Bowlby's attachment theory (Bowlby 1969) is an adaptationist model that attempts to explain how what seem to be irrational behaviors, such as phobias, could be exaggerated versions of normal fears that could have had a value in the "environment of evolutionary adaptiveness." According to this model, because human beings evolved as hunter-gatherers, their genes were molded to produce behaviors that were most useful under those conditions, and there has not been enough time for further evolution to take place since the relatively recent dawn of civilization. It is possible that variations in levels of fear and propensities to take action under stress represented different adaptive possibilities in such environments.

This adaptationist argument could be applied to some of the specific behaviors related to the impulsive dimension of BPD. Some behaviors that appear to be dysfunctional may serve a biological purpose. For example, some of the sexual impulsivity in female borderline patients could be adaptive in social environments where males are less reliable as providers. This "r strategy" involves earlier and more frequent reproduction (Wilson 1975) and could compensate for the lack of male support. There is in fact some evidence that in the absence of a father, young women reach puberty and become sexually active at an earlier age (Belsky et al. 1991).

Of course there is nothing adaptive about the overtly self-destructive symptoms seen in BPD. There are two possible explanations. One is that maladaptive behaviors can be linked to adaptive ones genetically, an example of a phenomenon called *pleiotropy*. The other, which will be proposed in this book, is that self-destructive behaviors result from environmentally determined but pathological amplifications of impulsive personality traits.

Affective instability is another trait that need not always be maladaptive. It is possible that there are normal variations in emotional lability, different levels of which could be adaptive or maladaptive depending on environmental considerations. It has been argued (Bowlby 1969) that the mood change in depression as a response to loss is potentially adaptive because it evokes comforting responses from significant others. The affective lability seen in borderline patients can also evoke social reinforcements, and its pathological aspect is an inability to modulate this emotionality when environmental circumstances make doing so a requirement.

Similar theoretical arguments could be used to account for other personality traits. Meehl (1990) has suggested that a schizotypal trait is much more widely distributed than the disorders with which it is associated (schizophrenia and schizotypal personality), and that this trait by itself need not decrease reproductive capacity. This line of reasoning could explain why the biological vulnerability for schizophrenia has not been eliminated from the gene pool.

Anxiety-related traits, which are predominant in Cluster C personality disorders, could also be a product of an extreme range of genetic variability. Studies have noted a hereditary factor in Axis I anxiety disorders (Barlow 1988), and research into social anxiety in childhood (Kagan et al. 1988) has demonstrated a strong genetic factor in shyness. Greater degrees of interpersonal anxiety could be adaptive in environments where strangers represent a potential physical danger. However, such traits, when amplified, could interfere with reproductive capacity.

An adaptationist approach can help clarify the dimensions of personality described in Chapter 2. For example, in Cloninger's schema, novelty seeking, harm avoidance, and reward dependence all represent behaviors that could be normative and potentially adaptive. It is only at levels beyond the normal ranges of variation, and when more than one dimension is abnormal, that there is an increased risk for overt psychopathology.

In summary, an adaptationist approach sheds light on the relationship of personality traits to personality disorders. Traits, which show such strong heritability, would not remain in the gene pool if they were not potentially adaptive. But when traits are amplified to become disorders, they in most cases interfere with fertility. In fact, it has been shown that patients with BPD have few children (Stone 1990). But at the trait level, the biological risk factors for BPD would not interfere with reproduction.

Evidence for Biological Vulnerability in Borderline Personality Disorder

Because heritability is associated more with traits than with disorders, we are still left with the question of whether patients with BPD have a demonstrable biological vulnerability. There are a number of methodological approaches that have been taken to investigate this problem.

One approach involves studies that attempt to determine whether BPD has a genetic pattern of inheritance. The methods involve family pedigree studies, twin studies, and adoption studies. The strongest finding of family pedigree studies (Zanarini 1993a) is that the relatives of borderline patients are more likely to have other impulse spectrum disorders, such as ASPD or substance abuse. There is also a greater frequency of affective disorders, but only in the relatives of borderline patients with comorbid depression. One study examined personality traits in the relatives of BPD probands (Silverman et al. 1991) and found that these traits were characterized by either impulsivity or affective instability, the core dimensions of BPD. Although most BPD probands do not have a relative with the disorder, there is a greater frequency of BPD in relatives than in comparison groups (Links et al. 1990a). None of the pedigree studies found any specific pattern of inheritance. In any case, this method cannot separate genetic from environmental influences.

The only twin study of BPD, done by Torgersen (1984), did not show monozygotic-dizygotic differences, although the number of subjects was far too small for any firm conclusion to be made. Since the publication of his paper, Torgersen (personal communication, 1991) has studied 25 monozygotic twin pairs, only 2 of which were concordant. There have been no adoption studies of BPD, although such studies would be quite feasible, since borderline patients are among the most likely groups of patients to give up their children for adoption (van Reekum et al. 1993).

The overall findings from the genetic studies of BPD, therefore, do not show that the disorder is heritable. In this respect, BPD is no different from the other Axis II diagnoses (McGuffin and Thapar 1992).

A second approach to the biological factors in BPD involves studies of biological markers. It should be noted that such markers, when found, do not necessarily demonstrate a biological etiological factor and may, in fact, reflect pathogenesis. In fact, no specific biological risk factors have been found in BPD. For example, markers associated with depression, such as abnormal dexamethasone suppression or decreased REM latency, appear only in those borderline patients who are also depressed (Gunderson and Phillips 1991).

Markers for trait impulsivity are somewhat more specific. Coccaro et al. (1989) compared personality disorders and affective disorders by examining serotonin activity as measured by the fenfluramine challenge test. There was a significant flattening of the response in BPD patients, which reflects a sluggishness in serotonin activity. The differences were much clearer when traits rather than disorders were considered, and serotonin activity was particularly low in patients with high scores for impulsive aggression on psychological tests. This study was carried out on a small group of male veterans, which is not a typical population of borderline patients. However, similar results have been found in a small sample of subjects from our own study of females with BPD (Martial et al. 1993). But in another study of serotonin activity in BPD (D. L. Gardner et al. 1990), levels of the serotonin metabolite 5-hydroxyindoleacetic acid (5-HIAA) in cerebrospinal fluid did not differ between BPD patients and control subjects except when the borderline patients had a history of suicide attempts. This is another example of how biological markers relate more strongly to behaviors than to diagnoses.

One problem with strictly neurochemical theories of mental disorders is that they do not take into account organization on the neurophysiological level. Although changes that are specific to the major psychiatric illnesses have not generally been found using electroencephalography, more sophisticated ways to use this technique have been developed. One of them, the P300, reflects brain activity in response to a new stimulus. Kutcher et al. (1987) examined this marker in BPD and found abnormal responses that resembled those seen in schizophrenia.

Recent technological advances, such as positron-emission tomography (PET), allow one to examine brain activity in detail and in vivo. So far there has been one report of PET scan results in a small sample of patients (Goyer et al. 1991), in which reduced activity in the frontal and parietal lobes was found in BPD subjects. The strongest relationships were between brain activity and an aggression scale, again showing that biological findings relate more to traits than to disorders.

Another approach to measuring neurophysiological changes in mental disorders is neuropsychological testing. A number of studies reviewed by van Reekum et al. (1993), most particularly the work of Andrulonis et al. (1982), have suggested that borderline patients show "soft" neurological signs. Most of these studies were done on male patients, some of whom also had a history of head injury, and it is not clear if these observations relate to etiological factors in BPD. It has been theorized, nonetheless, that the behavioral abnormalities of borderline patients suggest abnormalities in limbic activity and/or cortical modulation of the limbic system (Stone 1993a). One report (O'Leary et al. 1991) also suggested that some of the clinical features in BPD could be associated with problems in the recall of complex learned material and that this deficit could be reversed by cueing (a procedure that resembles the structuring techniques in therapy to be discussed in Chapters 8 and 9).

We can summarize as equivocal the findings from all the methods by which biological factors in BPD have been investigated. The studies of neurotransmitter activity that are linked to Siever's psychobiological theory of the personality disorders may be the most heuristic for further research. We will therefore examine Siever's theoretical structure in some detail.

Neurotransmitters and Personality Disorders

The theoretical model of Siever (Siever and Davis 1991) links the activity of neurotransmitter systems both to personality traits and to personality disorders. Each of four systems (mood-affect, impulse-action, attention-cognition, and anxiety) is linked to mental disorders on Axes I and II and is associated with specific biological markers.

The mood-affect system is associated with affective disorders on Axis I but partly accounts for the phenomenology of the dramatic cluster on Axis II, including BPD. The neurotransmitter that is involved is norepinephrine, which is associated with behavioral activation. However, there are important differences between the biology of mood in the affective disorders and that of the affective instability in the dramatic cluster personality disorders. The qualitative distinction between mood in BPD and in the affective disorders is based on the degree of environmental responsiveness in borderline patients (Gunderson and Phillips 1991). Siever and Davis (1991) have suggested that this hyperresponsiveness to the interpersonal environment reflects defects in modulation by the cholinergic system.

There is support for this model of the role of norepinephine from earlier studies in which catecholamine activity was linked to impulsivity (Gurrera 1990), and, when platelet MAO activity was used as a biological marker, to extraversion and novelty seeking (Zuckerman 1979). These traits have also been measured in studies of cortical evoked potentials, in which an "augmenting" response reflects stimulus seeking, whereas a "reducing" response reflects a damping down of responsiveness when stimuli are presented (Buchsbaum 1974). Southwick et al. (1990) have found some evidence for alterations in adrenergic receptors in BPD.

The impulse-action system is associated with impulse disorders on Axis I and with BPD or ASPD on Axis II. The neurotransmitter that is involved is serotonin, which is associated with behavioral inhibition. If serotonin functions as "the brakes," reductions in serotonin activity would lead to an inability to stop behavioral responses and to an increase in impulsivity and aggressivity. There is support for this concept of the role of serotonin from earlier studies (Åsberg et al. 1976; G. L. Brown et al. 1979), which have shown that the level of the serotonin metabolite 5-HIAA in cerebrospinal fluid relates to impulsive aggressiveness as well as to violent methods of suicide.

The attention-cognition system is linked to schizophrenia and to personality disorders in the schizophrenic spectrum. The anxiety system would be linked to the anxiety disorders and to the anxious cluster personality disorders.

In Siever's model it is the interaction of abnormalities in multiple systems that increases the risk for personality disorders. BPD could involve a combined dysfunction, with serotonin being less active and norepinephrine being overactive. Abnormal levels of activation without behavioral inhibition might be the kind of combination that could raise the risk of borderline psychopathology (Coccaro 1991). Neurotransmitter activity would distinguish dramatic cluster disorders such as BPD from anxious cluster disorders such as avoidant personality disorder, in which affective instability is associated with anxiety rather than impulsivity, or from odd cluster disorders such as schizotypal personality disorder.

No doubt these theories will be found to be too simple. As discussed in the last chapter, there are multiple receptors and multiple systems associated with each neurotransmitter. Nevertheless, it is within the realm of possibility that this research will eventually be able to pinpoint biological markers that are specific to the traits that underlie BPD and the other impulse spectrum disorders.

Biological Factors and the Core Dimensions of Borderline Personality Disorder

Because Siever's theory is concordant with the findings of phenomeno-logical studies that impulsivity and affective instability are the core dimensions of BPD, the working hypothesis of this book is that these dimensions could be the heritable traits behind BPD. Both dimensions would have to be abnormal, and the interactions between them could form a negative feedback loop. Affective instability leads to impulsive action to relieve dysphoria, and impulsive actions lead to negative con-sequences that feed affective instability.

Linehan (1987, 1993; Linehan and Koerner 1993) has developed a theory that takes these biological factors into account. She describes the biological risk factor in BPD as "emotional vulnerability." By this she means primarily affective instability, in that borderline patients are ex-cessively sensitive to emotional input and have intense and protracted reactions to even low levels of stimulation. A contrasting view comes from a recent study by Torgersen (1993), who found that impulsive symptoms were more heritable, whereas affective ones related more to the shared environment (i.e., the family).

The cognitive symptoms associated with BPD do not fall under the core dimensions and may have entirely different biological roots. To the extent that such symptoms resemble those seen in schizophrenia, one might wish to investigate the dopaminergic system in borderline pa-tients. However, it is also possible that these phenomena, which are not associated with fixed delusions, are dissociative in nature. As will be discussed in Chapter 4, patients with BPD have a high level of dissocia-tive phenomena (Zweig-Frank et al., in press). The capacity to dissoci-ate may itself reflect a biological variability that is independent of the core dimensions.

It will take a good deal more research to determine whether one or both of the core dimensions reflect the biological factors in BPD. Be-cause the widest variety of evidence supports the biological nature of impulsivity and affective instability, the theoretical structure of this book assumes that both dimensions are required for BPD to develop.

It is likely that personality disorders are more complex than can be accounted for by a few simple dimensions (Kagan 1993; Siever 1993). As discussed in Chapter 2, only the categorical construct of BPD captures the uniqueness of this population. However, biological dimensions could shed light on the interaction of biological and other risk factors in BPD. Siever's theory is sufficiently heuristic to justify using it as the provisional basis of a multidimensional approach to BPD.

Summary

The evidence presented in this chapter points to personality traits as the underlying heritable factors behind personality disorders. It is therefore not surprising that the evidence for specific biological markers in BPD has been weak. It remains possible that future technologies will elicit stronger findings, but these findings will most likely continue to be associated with traits.

The argument of this chapter is that biological risk factors are necessary but not sufficient for the development of borderline pathology. Without them, even the worst environment will produce a different disorder. With them, environmental risk factors will be required for the emergence of the full disorder.

Linehan (1993) has also developed a theory in which constitutional factors interact with psychological risk factors. She hypothesizes an interaction between an "emotional vulnerability" and an "invalidating parental environment." A similar view of the interaction of biological and psychological risks in BPD will be presented in Chapter 6. In the next chapter we examine psychological factors that may also be necessary but not sufficient risks for BPD.

4

Psychological Risk Factors

T here is quite a bit of evidence that psychological factors play a role in the development of borderline personality disorder. The risk factors are related to a variety of childhood experiences and fall into three general categories: trauma, early separation or loss, and abnormal parenting. Individual borderline patients may show a predominance of one risk factor or all three together. Although trauma appears to be somewhat more specific to BPD, none of the risk factors is specific enough to draw any firm conclusions about its etiological role. There are many individuals with the same experiences who have other disorders or no disorder. Therefore, like biological vulnerability, psychological risk factors are necessary but not sufficient conditions for developing BPD.

Methodological Issues in Measuring Psychological Risk Factors

Most of the research that will be discussed in this chapter involves the measurement of psychological risk factors through retrospective designs. But simply asking patients to remember their childhood experiences raises questions of validity. No one can be sure whether adult memories of childhood are really accurate, because such memories can later become distorted and because problems in later life often color perceptions of childhood. In particular, there has been a good deal of concern recently that therapists who are convinced by trauma theories are eliciting false memories of child abuse in suggestible patients (Loftus 1993). In fact, the theory that traumatic experiences in childhood can be entirely repressed for many years is quite controversial and is not in accord with the intrusive qualities of memories seen in posttraumatic stress disorder (PTSD) (Loftus 1993).

Personality disorders could be another source of inaccuracy in how patients retrospectively view their childhood experiences. Because borderline patients tend to have distorted perceptions of their relationships in adulthood, their memories of childhood could be equally unreliable. Ideally, such perceptions would require some form of independent validation. At the very least, researchers need to take special precautions with personality disorder patients, preferably accepting only clear and detailed memories that have not been subject to "repression."

Ideally, the most valid way to study psychological risk factors is in prospective designs. For example, if a cohort of children were followed longitudinally into adulthood, we could use independent observations of their experiences and relationships with their families to predict which of them would develop psychopathology. In view of the practical problems of conducting this kind of research, investigators have had to accept the limitations of retrospective designs. But in a recent review, Brewin et al. (1993) concluded that given the possibility of independently validating reports of childhood experience, the limitations of retrospective designs have been exaggerated. For example, L. N. Robins et al. (1985) found that siblings give highly concordant reports about the factual aspects of childhood experiences. Reports of incestuous childhood sexual abuse were found, by Herman and Schatzow (1987), to be verifiable through siblings, although this study was not repeated in nonincestuous cases. The validity of instruments that measure nonfactual variables such as family atmosphere is less well established, and in the Robins et al. study there was little sibling concordance for measures based on perceptions of the quality of family life. One possible exception could be the Parental Bonding Index (PBI; Parker 1981), an instrument that measures perceptions of parent-child relationships and that has been adequately validated both by sibling concordance and by the relationship of abnormal scores to a number of psychiatric diagnoses (Parker 1983).

Nevertheless, the retrospective nature of the research to be discussed in this chapter remains a limitation, and all of the findings that will be discussed should ultimately be confirmed by prospective studies. What we can say at this point is that the research findings on psychological risk factors in BPD are coherent and fairly consistent.

The Role of Trauma

The concept that traumatic experiences in childhood can produce mental disorders in adulthood was one of the early ideas behind psychoanalysis. As theories of psychopathology became more complex, it was no longer assumed that early traumatic events have a linear relationship to adult dysfunction. In psychoanalysis, the intrapsychic elaboration of experience came to be seen as more important than the actual events of early life. Cognitive-behavioral theory has also emphasized the importance of the processing of life experience (Beck and Freeman 1990). Theories derived from family therapy have suggested that psychopathology is based on subtle but enduring factors, such as long-lasting structural abnormalities in family life (Lewis et al. 1976).

The return of trauma to a central position in psychiatry was related to a number of political and social events that influenced the psychiatric zeitgeist. The inclusion of PTSD in the DSM-III (American Psychiatric Association 1980) may have been a response to the experience of psychiatrists treating war veterans who were experiencing long-lasting effects of earlier traumatic events (Kelley 1985). Although the extent to which the psychopathology seen in veterans could be attributed to pre-existing personality disturbance rather than war trauma is unclear, the concept of PTSD met a felt need.

In understanding the recent interest in the role of trauma in producing psychopathology, it is also useful to consider the profound impact that feminist theory has had on psychiatry. Feminist-inspired research has played a crucial role in studying the frequency and long-term effects of child abuse (Russell 1986) and in demonstrating the frequency of abuse experiences in the personality disorders (Herman 1992). Feminist theory emphasizes the psychosocial factors in mental disorders, particularly effects deriving from the oppression of women. Therefore, conditions that are more common in women are of particular importance for these researchers. A high percentage of individuals diagnosed with BPD are females, and it has been hypothesized that this gender difference might be due to the more frequent sexual abuse of female children (Stone 1990).

Trauma has also been proposed as a general explanation for the etiology of BPD (Herman and van der Kolk 1987). In this theory, intense trauma, particularly if repressed, could produce a chronic posttraumatic disorder that affects the entire personality. There are a number of reasons to be cautious about this hypothesis. First, a PTSD model does not account for the full range of borderline phenomenology (Gunderson and Sabo 1993). Second, as we will see in this chapter, the relationship between childhood experiences and BPD is complex, and the pathway from traumatic events to adult psychopathology may not be mediated by posttraumatic mechanisms. Although the posttraumatic theory of BPD has stimulated a great deal of research, it is unidimensional and overly simplifies a complex process (Paris and Zweig-Frank 1992).

Even in the most severe cases of trauma, there are interactions with underlying personality traits that determine how the trauma is processed and what its long-term consequences will be (Horowitz 1976; Sigal and Weinfeld 1989). To put the problem in perspective, we need to look beyond the incidence of trauma in clinical populations and examine its effect in nonpatients. The largest research literature on the effects of traumatic experiences in community populations is on childhood sexual abuse.

Childhood Sexual Abuse

Long-Term Effects and the Parameters of Abuse

Childhood sexual abuse has been shown to produce a number of long-term effects in adult life (Browne and Finkelhor 1986). Some of the difficulties that occur more frequently in individuals with histories of childhood sexual abuse include depression, suicide attempts, substance abuse, revictimization, and problems with intimate relationships. It should not escape notice that these are among the predominant symptoms of the borderline personality. However, most victims of sexual abuse do not show these features. As a matter of fact, only about 20% of childhood sexual abuse survivors have any measurable psychopathology (Browne and Finkelhor 1986). Only a small percentage are likely to have a diagnosable personality disorder.

It is therefore crucial to determine the mechanisms by which abuse does lead to psychopathology. A major literature review by Browne and Finkelhor (1986) shows that we cannot understand the effects of childhood sexual abuse without considering its nature, that is, the parameters of abuse. These parameters include the frequency of abusive events, the duration of the abusive relationship, the relationship of the child to the perpetrator, the age of the child at the onset of the abuse, the age of the offender, the type of sexual act, whether force was used, whether there was disclosure, and what the parental reaction was to that disclosure. Each of these parameters could be a more powerful predictor of outcome than the fact of abuse alone. Studies of sexual abuse in clinical populations that fail to take this into account and simply count the number of patients who have had some sort of abusive experience are missing a crucial interaction point in the causal link to psychopathology. It is therefore worthwhile to consider each of these parameters separately.

It should be noted that all the community studies of the effects of childhood sexual abuse are retrospective. We lack prospective studies of abused children in the community, and such research would be a better way to determine which parameters are most relevant to long-term outcome. Nevertheless, the existing retrospective community studies can shed important light on the potential role of childhood sexual abuse in BPD. Unless stated otherwise, all of the conclusions discussed below are drawn from Browne and Finkelhor (1986).

Frequency and Duration

It seems self-evident that the more frequently any traumatic event occurs, the more likely it is to produce long-term effects. Several studies have shown that this is the case for childhood sexual abuse. Peters (1988) found frequency and duration to be the most powerful predictors in a regression on global psychopathology. But Peters also found that most reports of childhood sexual abuse in her community study were in fact single events. Such incidents are unlikely to produce long-lasting effects.

Severity

The severity of the event is of crucial importance in the long-term outcome of sexual abuse. Children who have been subjected to sexual abuse involving penetration are the most damaged. Researchers and clinicians must be careful to distinguish between sexual abuse and psychologically abusive situations, and should not consider noncontact experiences, such as exhibitionism, verbal threats, or inappropriately sexualized relationships, in the same category as childhood sexual abuse. In taking into account how intrusive the abuse really was, one needs to separate out fondling, genital fondling, oral sex, and most particularly penetration. In addition, because the use of force has been found to be one of the most powerful predictors of long-term outcome, it needs to be determined whether violence or more subtle methods of persuasion were applied to the child.

Relation to the Perpetrator

The child's relation to the perpetrator has been found in many studies to be the most important determinant of the outcome of childhood sexual abuse. In particular, abuse from a caregiver is more pathogenic. There are also important differences depending on which family member is the perpetrator. One of the most robust findings in the literature is that father-daughter incest is the most pathogenic form of childhood sexual abuse. However, father-daughter pairs account for a minority of incest reports (Finkelhor et el. 1990; Russell 1986), the majority of which involve abuse by stepfathers, uncles, cousins, and siblings. It is obviously important that researchers not bracket together childhood sexual abuse events from different perpetrators.

There is a crucial psychological difference between intrafamilial abuse (incest) and extrafamilial abuse (molestation). It makes perfect sense that researchers have found incest to be more associated with psychopathology, because it is a betrayal—a use of one's body by family members whom one needs to trust for protection. The impact of incest can only be understood in terms of that betrayal of trust and of the pathological dynamics of the incest family. Sexual molestation by strangers is less traumatic and may also reflect the effects of preexisting family pathology. In one study (Fromuth 1986), the impact of molestation on adult psychopathology disappeared in multivariate analysis when a measure of maternal warmth was added.

Age at Onset
The effects of childhood sexual abuse can be influenced by the age at which it begins. Sexual abuse is most common in latency, but the earlier it starts, the worse the long-term outcome. The effects also depend on the age difference between the victim and the perpetrator. We need to be careful not to consider as childhood sexual abuse incidents of consenting sexual activity involving early adolescents.

Disclosure
The long-term effects of childhood sexual abuse can be mediated by whether the incident is disclosed, whether there is an appropriate response to that disclosure, and whether action is taken to prevent repetition. Many of the traumatic effects of sexual abuse during childhood are due to the secrecy of the event and to the child's perception that even if she were to ask her mother for help, she either would not be believed or would not get a helpful response. However, disclosure can also lead to negative effects, especially if it results in family breakdown (Sauzier 1989).

Childhood Sexual Abuse in the Community

The prevalence of childhood sexual abuse in the community varies widely from one study to another. These discrepancies are quite serious, with the rates varying from 6% to 54% in various reports (Finkelhor 1986). Some of this variability can be accounted for by methodological issues such as the definition of childhood sexual abuse used, as well as how many questions were used and whether they were asked in a face-to-face interview. A national survey of sexual abuse in the United States showed that there are also genuine population differences for rates of childhood sexual abuse in different communities (Finkelhor et al. 1990).

Nevertheless, the best studies offer a fairly coherent picture of the prevalence of childhood sexual abuse. A national study in the United States (Finkelhor et al. 1990) found that 27% of women and 16% of men reported some form of sexual abuse. The median age at which the abuse occurred was between 9 and 10 years for both sexes. In both sexes the perpetrators were almost all males, and most of the perpetrators were either strangers or nonrelatives. Incest accounted for about 5% of cases in females and was not found in males; if a relative was a perpetrator, it was most likely to be an uncle or a cousin. The vast majority of reports were of single incidents. A minority of cases involved penetration or force. A well-conducted national Canadian study (Committee on Sexual Offences Against Children and Youth, Canada 1984) reported similar findings: 25% of females under age 16 had experienced some kind of sexual offense, but only half of these incidents involved contact. Among the 12% of women who had experienced childhood sexual abuse, incestuous abuse from a relative before age 16 accounted for only a quarter (i.e., 3% of the total sample) of all incidents. Higher rates of childhood sexual abuse have been obtained in two other well-designed studies (Russell 1986; Wyatt 1985), and the discrepancy between studies might be explained by regional differences. Both Russell and Wyatt conducted their surveys in California, and Finkelhor et al. (1990) found much higher rates of childhood sexual abuse in California (not in those individuals who had been brought up there, but in those who had moved there from other parts of the country).

The overall rate of sexual abuse in the community, or of severe sexual abuse, is clearly much greater than the prevalence of BPD. Based on interview data from the Epidemiologic Catchment Area study, Swartz et al. (1990) suggested that the prevalence of BPD is about 2%. This prevalence was about the same in two other studies that used self-report instruments (Reich et al. 1989; Ross 1991). Clearly childhood sexual abuse by itself does not necessarily lead to BPD. Either other risk factors are required or else only some forms of sexual abuse produce this form of psychopathology. It is therefore worth examining in some detail the evidence that links abuse with borderline pathology.

Childhood Sexual Abuse and Borderline Personality Disorder

A number of the long-term effects of childhood sexual abuse resemble borderline pathology. There are now findings from a number of centers which show that borderline patients have a particularly high frequency of childhood sexual abuse compared with groups of nonborderline patients. Nine empirical studies (Briere and Zaidi 1989; Byrne et al. 1990; Herman et al. 1989; Links et al. 1988b; Ludolph et al. 1990; Ogata et al. 1990b; Shearer et al. 1990; Westen et al. 1990; Zanarini et al. 1989b) have shown that childhood sexual abuse is frequent in BPD. The overall rate in most reports was about 70%, which was significantly greater than the rates found in any of the control groups.

However, there are problems with most of these studies. First, few researchers have systematically examined the parameters of sexual abuse in BPD. Of the nine studies, abuse was considered as a single variable in five of them. Only two studies (Links et al. 1988b; Zanarini et al. 1989b) separated the perpetrators of childhood sexual abuse into caretakers and noncaretakers, and only two studies (Ogata et al. 1990b; Westen et al. 1990) examined the relation of the perpetrator to the abused child. Second, sexual abuse could intercorrelate with other psychological risk factors for BPD, a possibility that most of the nine studies did not examine.

There was clearly a need for a large-scale study of abuse in BPD in which all the abuse parameters were examined and in which abuse and other psychological risk factors were examined multivariately. Such a study has recently been completed by a research team in which the author was a principal investigator. Much of the discussion to follow will derive from this research, which was designed and carried out by the author and Dr. Hallie Zweig-Frank. This is the first study to have examined in detail the nature of the relationship between childhood sexual abuse and BPD by measuring all the parameters described in the childhood sexual abuse literature and by examining sexual abuse multi-variately along with a wide range of other psychological risk factors. In addition, the specificity of childhood sexual abuse to BPD was put to a critical test by using a control group of individuals with personality disorders other than BPD. The analysis of the results of this project have recently been completed (Paris et al. 1994a), and the results reported below are derived from this analysis.

Because the frequency of childhood sexual abuse is much higher in women (Jason et al. 1982), and because the risk factors might differ by gender, the first stage of the study was carried out on female subjects only. The second stage involved repeating the study on male subjects.

The female sample consisted of 150 women between the ages of 18 and 48 with a diagnosis of personality disorder (Paris et al. 1994a). Using the Diagnostic Interview for Borderlines, Revised, the subjects were divided into a BPD group of 78 and a non-BPD group of 72. The majority of the subjects in the nonborderline group had either Axis II Cluster C disorders or nonspecified personality disorders, generally with a mixture of traits from several Cluster C categories. The childhood histories were evaluated with another semistructured interview conducted by an experienced child psychiatrist (Dr. Jaswant Guzder), who was blind to diagnosis. Particular care was taken in these interviews not to accept as valid memories that were either vague or else produced in therapy or under hypnosis.

The frequency of childhood sexual abuse in women with BPD (71%) was found to be significantly higher than in the non-BPD group (46%). However, because nearly half the nonborderline subjects also had childhood sexual abuse, a history of sexual abuse only made it 1.5 times more likely that the personality disorder diagnosis for any subject would be BPD. Therefore, we examined the childhood sexual abuse parameters to take a closer look at the relationship between abuse histories and borderline psychopathology.

In the community studies, relation to the perpetrator had been of particular importance for understanding the effects of childhood sexual abuse. But we found that there were no differences between the BPD and non-BPD samples for rates of childhood sexual abuse from any of their caregivers (father, mother, stepfather, stepmother). Abuse by a caregiver did not, in fact, constitute the majority of childhood sexual abuse reports, and the overall rate for childhood sexual abuse from any caregiver in BPD was 26%, almost exactly the same percentage obtained in two other studies (Links et al. 1988; Zanarini et al. 1989b). The widely reported frequencies of 70% for childhood sexual abuse in BPD could be misleading if childhood sexual abuse were to be confused with incest. In fact, father-daughter incest only occurred in about 15% of subjects from each of our groups. We found that, in confirmation of another study that examined specific perpetrators (Ogata et al. 1990b), the higher overall rate of childhood sexual abuse in BPD is accounted for by incidents of molestation by nonfamily members such as neighbors or strangers or by incestuous abuse from other family members such as uncles, cousins, and grandparents.

Community studies had also shown that the effects of childhood sexual abuse from any perpetrator are more severe if the incidents were frequent, if the abusive relationship lasted for a long time, if the child was younger when the abuse started, if penetration occurred, if force was used, and if the child could not tell anyone or get help. Our study examined all of these parameters and found that in the majority of abused subjects from both groups, childhood sexual abuse occurred during latency, was accompanied by the use of force, and was not disclosed, and help was not obtained at the time of the incident. However, none of these parameters discriminated borderline subjects with childhood sexual abuse from nonborderline subjects with childhood sexual abuse. In both groups, frequency and duration showed a bimodal distribution such that, although some subjects reported long-term abuse, the greatest number of childhood sexual abuse events (80%) involved single incidents. Given that abuse of greater frequency and duration is more likely to lead to psychopathology, this finding sheds doubt on the overall etiological significance of childhood sexual abuse in BPD.

The one parameter in our study that discriminated abused BPD subjects from abused non-BPD subjects was the severity of sexual abuse: 30% of the abused BPD subjects (about a quarter of the total sample) but only 6% of the abused non-BPD subjects had experienced childhood sexual abuse with penetration, a highly significant difference. Therefore, penetration, a more traumatic type of abuse, increased the risk for developing BPD. These findings have recently been confirmed in another study (Silk et al. 1993).

We also found that 37% of the abused BPD group but only 14% of the abused non-BPD group had suffered childhood sexual abuse from multiple perpetrators. This finding has also recently been confirmed by Silk et al. (1993). There are several possible explanations for this difference: 1) that children who develop BPD have a high exposure to trauma; 2) that once traumatized, these children are susceptible to revictimization; or 3) that there is some other factor in these children that makes them susceptible to becoming abused.

The second phase of the project involved examining a sample of 121 male subjects (Paris et al. 1994b). Of these subjects, 61 had BPD and 60 had personality disorders other than BPD (again mostly in Cluster C). Because, as noted above, community studies had shown that sexual abuse is less common in males (Jason et al. 1982), we did not expect to find high rates in males with BPD. But the results were in fact rather similar to those in the female sample. As many as 45% of the BPD patients had a history of childhood sexual abuse, as opposed to 25% of the non-BPD subjects, which was a significant difference. The sexual abuse was almost entirely homosexual, and most of the perpetrators were relatives outside the nuclear family or else strangers. Although as in the females, the vast majority of reports were again of single incidents, the childhood sexual abuse parameters that distinguished the two diagnostic groups were penetration and the use of force.

Our findings would therefore suggest that childhood sexual abuse is a risk factor for BPD in both males and females. However, many of the findings of our research are not consistent with a posttraumatic theory of the etiology of BPD. The large overlap between the rates of childhood sexual abuse for borderline and nonborderline personality disorders indicates that sexual abuse has a low specificity in relation to BPD. When we consider the childhood sexual abuse parameters, the perpetrators were not in most cases caregivers, who have been associated with a more severe outcome. One of the most striking findings was the high rate of single incidents, which, as shown in community studies, are much less likely to be associated with psychopathology. Severe abuse, as measured by penetration and multiple perpetration, was what most clearly discriminated BPD patients, but it occurred in only a minority of the cases.

To summarize the results, childhood sexual abuse was found to be common in BPD patients. However, not all BPD patients had a history of childhood sexual abuse, and many non-BPD patients, as well as non-patients, also had such histories. Moreover, those BPD patients with childhood sexual abuse were found to have had a variety of experiences, some more and some less traumatic. Finally, it seems that the more severe the childhood sexual abuse, the higher the risk for BPD.

It is in the subgroup of BPD patients with severe abuse that childhood sexual abuse may be particularly important. If we had excluded from the analysis the subjects who reported childhood sexual abuse with penetration, the overall rates of sexual abuse in the BPD and non-BPD samples would have been virtually identical. Our findings parallel the results of multivariate community studies presented earlier which found that penetration was the single most powerful predictor of psychopathology in adults with childhood sexual abuse.

The Link Between Childhood Sexual Abuse and
Borderline Personality Disorder: Possible Mechanisms

One possible explanation of the lack of specificity for childhood sexual abuse in BPD is that childhood experiences have a different impact depending on how they are processed by the individual (Rutter and Rutter 1993). For example, Finkelhor (1988) suggests that the long-term effects of childhood sexual abuse cannot be adequately explained solely by posttraumatic mechanisms but also require cognitive changes, including sexualization, betrayal, stigmatization, and powerlessness. Individual differences in cognitive processing could explain why even severe childhood sexual abuse is not consistently related to adult psychopathology. These differences might depend on variability in personality traits.

Childhood sexual abuse also interacts with other psychological risk factors, and these interactions, as well as the trauma itself, could influence whether childhood sexual abuse leads to severe psychopathology. There is evidence that sexual abuse is associated with a pathological family atmosphere. For example, in one recent study (Nash et al. 1993), the long-term effects of childhood sexual abuse in both clinical and community populations were shown to be dependent on abnormalities in family functioning. In the national survey of childhood sexual abuse discussed earlier, Finkelhor et al. (1990) also found a strong relationship between abuse histories and reports of serious family dysfunction.

In incest cases, important areas of family dysfunction have been described that accompany the incestuous event (Courtois 1988). Some researchers have suggested that the pathological dynamics of incest families could be as important as the trauma of the incestuous event (Burgess and Conger 1978). The same consideration applies to understanding the phenomenon of extrafamilial molestation. Children who are neglected by their families could be more susceptible to becoming molested; they are lonely and vulnerable and may not be able to protect their boundaries when approached by perpetrators. A study of pedophiles (Conte et al. 1989) found that these individuals were able to recognize potential victims by their obvious vulnerability and to approach them selectively.

To study the interaction of childhood sexual abuse and other psychological risk factors in BPD, we need to measure whether these factors also increase the risk for BPD. The empirical findings concerning the role of other forms of trauma, as well as separation or loss, and abnormalities in parenting will be discussed below. In addition, multivariate research that examines all the risk factors together will be discussed at the end of this chapter.

Are There Symptoms of Borderline Personality Disorder That Are Markers for Abuse?

There is some evidence that borderline patients who have experienced severe childhood sexual abuse are more symptomatic (Silk et al. 1993). But are there any characteristic symptoms that could identify this group in a clinical setting?

One suggestion has been that the presence of dissociation in BPD provides clues to a history of trauma (Herman and van der Kolk 1987). This link was based on evidence that dissociation is often associated with PTSD and on the theory that children learn to use this defense when overwhelmed by abusive experiences. In one recent study, there was a link between childhood sexual abuse and dissociative phenomena in both clinical and nonclinical populations, although this effect was found to be mediated by family pathology (Nash et al. 1993). There is evidence for some relationship between abuse and dissociation in female psychiatric populations (Chu and Dill 1990) as well as in borderline patients (Herman et al. 1989; Ogata et al. 1990b).

In our own study, we found that scores on a standard measure, the Dissociative Experiences Scale (DES; Bernstein and Putnam 1986), were twice as high in both female and male borderline patients than in patients with nonborderline personality disorders. Because dissociative symptoms and childhood sexual abuse both were more common in borderline patients, we examined the relationship between dissociation and childhood sexual abuse multivariately, taking diagnosis into account. In these analyses, dissociation had no relationship with sexual abuse or its parameters, or with any of the other psychological risk factors we studied (Zweig-Frank et al. 1994a, 1994b). (These results run counter to those of one previous study that had found an independent relationship between abuse and dissociation but that had not examined the parameters of abuse [Herman et al. 1989].) The absence of any link between dissociation and psychological risk factors was consistent in both female and male samples. This result led us to hypothesize that the capacity to dissociate could reflect not childhood experience, but some of the constitutional factors in BPD. We have recently found higher concordance for dissociative capacity in monozygotic as compared with dizygotic twins (J. Paris, H. Zweig-Frank, K. Jang, et al., manuscript submitted for publication).

Another symptom of BPD that has been theorized as being linked to histories of trauma is self-mutilation (Herman and van der Kolk 1987). It has been suggested that borderline patients mutilate themselves as a way of dealing with painful dissociative states (Leibenluft et al. 1987). One study (van der Kolk et al. 1991) found self-mutilation in BPD to be related both to a history of trauma and to dissociation. In our own research (Zweig-Frank et al. 1994a, 1994b), we found that self-mutilation was more common in both female and male BPD patients than in non-BPD patients, but that self-mutilation was not related to any of the psychological risk factors we measured. Although in univariate analysis self-mutilation was linked to higher levels of dissociation, this link was not found to be independent of diagnosis in multivariate analyses. Our findings also do not explain why some borderline patients mutilate themselves and others do not. The presence of self-mutilating symptoms might therefore reflect the impulsive dimension of borderline pathology rather than any particular life experience.

Another possible marker for abuse could be the defense styles seen in BPD patients. In our study we examined whether borderline patients use different defense mechanisms than do patients with other personality disorders. The essential finding was that in both the female and male samples, when defenses were measured by a standard self-report instrument, the Defense Style Questionnaire, subjects with BPD were found to have used more maladaptive defenses (Bond et al. 1994). But there was no relationship between defense style and histories of abuse, or between defense styles and any of the other psychological risk factors we studied. Defense style might therefore be another measure of the core dimensions of BPD and not of the psychological risk factors for the disorder.

One final possibility is that trauma in borderline patients might lead to a distinctive symptom profile. J. C. Perry (1991) and colleagues reported that in their study, borderline patients with trauma had more impulsive symptoms, whereas those with neglect had more affective symptoms. However, in a larger-scale study comparing abused and non-abused borderline patients, Zanarini et al. (1993) found no symptomatic differences between abused and nonabused patients with BPD.

On the whole, then, there are no clear-cut markers for abuse histories in BPD. The symptoms of borderline psychopathology seem to be about the same regardless of the individual weighting of psychological risk factors.

Physical Abuse, Family Violence, and Verbal Abuse in Borderline Personality Disorder

Physical abuse is a traumatic childhood experience that is known to increase the risk for adult psychopathology. As in sexual abuse, the long-term outcome of physical abuse depends on parameters such as frequency, duration, and severity (Malinosky-Rummell and Hansen 1993). Exposure to family violence, even when not directed at the child, may be a risk factor in its own right. Finally, verbal abuse of children by their parents may also predispose these children to later psychopathology.

The type of abuse suffered by children differs with gender. Epidemiological studies of community populations (Jason et al. 1982) have shown that whereas sexual abuse is much more common among females, physical abuse is more common among males. Rutter (1987) found that boys have more serious consequences than girls if exposed to family violence.

There are a number of lines of research which show that physical abuse can be associated with psychiatric disorders in adults. One study of male psychiatric outpatients (Swett et al. 1990) found that those patients with histories of physical abuse had more severe psychopathology. There is evidence from a large-scale prospective epidemiological study (Pollock et al. 1990) for an association of physical abuse with antisocial personality disorder (ASPD). In a study of psychiatric inpatients (G. R. Brown and Anderson 1991), men with histories of physical abuse were more likely to also abuse substances and/or be suicidal, two features of BPD. This finding suggests that physical abuse might be more important for the pathway to BPD in men than in women.

There are also a number of studies which show that physical abuse is common in the histories of borderline patients of both sexes (Herman et al. 1989; Shearer et al. 1990; Westen et al. 1990), although some researchers (Ogata et al. 1990b; Zanarini et al. 1989b) have not found these differences. In our study of female patients (Paris et al. 1994a), the rate of physical abuse was significantly greater in the BPD group than in the group with personality disorders other than BPD, with rates similar to those found for childhood sexual abuse (73% vs. 53%, respectively). As in the case of childhood sexual abuse, there was a good deal of overlap between our borderline and nonborderline samples for this risk factor. We examined several parameters of physical abuse, including frequency, duration, severity, and the abused child's relation to the perpetrator, but there were no differences between the female groups for any of these parameters. The results for the male sample were similar, with 66% of the BPD and 50% of the non-BPD subjects reporting physical abuse, a difference that statistically was only at trend level (Paris et al. 1994b). However, physical abuse from fathers was significantly more common in male borderline subjects, who also reported physical abuse of longer duration. As we concluded for sexual abuse, physical abuse may be a risk factor for BPD, but it is also associated with personality disorders in general.

There has been one study (Herman et al. 1989) in which borderline patients reported more frequent episodes in which they witnessed family violence. In another study (Zanarini et al. 1989b), verbal abuse was a surprisingly powerful correlate of borderline pathology. Although other forms of abuse are more dramatic, all of these factors could have profound effects on the self-esteem of a child, and they probably reflect a family atmosphere of uncontrolled hostility and threat. It may be that sexual, physical, and verbal abuse all have a similar impact on children. In fact, in the study of childhood experiences in BPD by Herman et al. (1989), the most significant differences from the control group were obtained by combining all forms of abuse into a "total trauma score."

Separation and Loss in Borderline Personality Disorder

There is evidence from four studies using differing methodologies (Bradley 1979; Paris et al. 1988; Soloff and Millward 1983a; Zanarini et al. 1989b) that borderline patients have a high frequency of early separation and loss from their parents during childhood. One study (Ogata et al. 1990a), however, did not confirm these differences. In all of these reports the control groups consisted of depressed patients. In our study of female subjects (Paris et al. 1994a), in which BPD patients were compared with patients with other personality disorders, a history of separation or loss before age 5 years was frequent (21%) in BPD, but no more so than in the control subjects. Separation or loss before age 16 was even more frequent (51%) in BPD, but again no more so than in other personality disorders. The results for the male sample (Paris et al. 1994b) were somewhat different in that there were significantly more separations or losses in BPD before age 16 (42.6%) than in the non-BPD comparison group; but the rate of separations or losses in male borderline patients before age 5 (16.4%) was no greater than in the non-BPD group.

Separation and loss probably constitute another important but non-specific psychological risk factor for BPD. A history of early separation and loss is not all that specific to any form of psychopathology and is seen with some frequency in normal populations (Tennant 1988). Lack of specificity does not mean that a risk factor does not play a role in the development of a mental disorder, but only that it does not by itself lead to that specific disorder. For example, the relationship of early loss to adult psychopathology has been shown to be influenced by a number of interacting factors, such as family dysfunction after the loss and buffering factors from outside the family (Rutter 1989; Tennant 1988). In interaction with other risk factors, separation and loss could still contribute to the development of BPD.

Parental Psychopathology and Borderline Personality Disorder

There are a number of lines of evidence which suggest that the parents of borderline patients have significant psychopathology. This pathology could manifest as overt psychiatric disorder or as personality traits that interfere with adequate performance of the tasks of parenting.

The most systematic study of psychiatric diagnoses in the parents of BPD patients was carried out by Links et al. (1988a). The parents of a cohort of borderline patients were either directly interviewed or assessed through data provided by another relative. The disorders with the greatest morbid risk in first-degree relatives were recurrent unipolar depression (27%), alcoholism (21%), BPD (15%), and ASPD (10%). These findings were in essential agreement with five other studies in which the parents were not directly examined (Baron et al. 1985; Loranger et al. 1982; Pope et al. 1983; Schulz et al. 1986; Soloff and Millward 1983b). It should not escape notice that most of the parental disorders were in the impulsive spectrum and that all of them suggest underlying deviations in impulsive and affective personality traits, as was found in a study by Silverman et al. (1991). Therefore, parental psychopathology may reflect, in part, common biological vulnerabilities that run in families. However, parental psychopathology of this kind seriously affects the quality of parenting. Parental alcoholism or either BPD or ASPD in a parent could be associated with trauma, neglect, or early separation and loss. Depression in a parent could also lead to emotional neglect of children.

Even in the absence of a psychiatric diagnosis, it is possible that the parents of borderline patients do not provide a sufficiently supportive environment for their children. There have been a few studies examining family structure in BPD patients. Gunderson et al. (1980), based on interviews with the families of young borderline inpatients, assessed the relationships between borderline patients and their families. These authors found that, compared with control groups, the parents of BPD patients were unresponsive and tended to scapegoat their child.

There have been studies that have used standard measurements of family functioning in BPD. Ogata et al. (1990a) assessed family functioning in adult borderline patients based on the Family Environment Scale, a standard measure of family experience. Compared with a control group of depressed patients, the BPD patients described significantly lower family cohesion. (Low cohesion implies that families are chaotic and have unclear boundaries.) Low family cohesion was also the main finding in a study of the children of borderline mothers (R. B. Feldman, P. Zelkowitz, M. Weiss, et al., manuscript submitted for publication). In one study (Silk et al. 1993), borderline patients with severe childhood sexual abuse had the least cohesive families among the groups studied. Low cohesion in families could also be associated with forms of trauma other than loss or with emotional neglect.

Parental Bonding in Borderline Personality Disorder

Attachment theory (Bowlby 1969, 1973, 1980) is an important theoretical framework for understanding the relationship between childhood experience and adult psychopathology. In this model, children are born with evolutionarily determined needs to attach to their parents, and when that attachment system breaks down, there are a number of psychological consequences. Secure attachment requires parental attitudes that are themselves secure and that communicate to the growing child a reliable parental presence as well as an expectation that when the child becomes autonomous, the parent will not withdraw. These key parental attitudes correspond to what developmental theorists (Rowe 1981) have defined as the "tasks of parenting." Essentially parents must provide sufficient emotional support to make children feel loved and secure, and then encourage them to become autonomous.

The absence of this emotional support provides an operational definition for emotional neglect. One consequence of such neglect can be that when parents fail to respond to emotional needs, children become dysphoric. Impulsive action can be an attempt to cope with intense and unmodulated negative affects. Insecure attachment to parents also leads to clinging behaviors (Bowlby 1973). Obviously some of the phenomena associated with anxious attachment are also characteristic of BPD.

It is on this basis that some clinicians working with borderline patients have suggested that disturbances in parenting, particularly a failure of parental responsiveness (Adler 1985), could be a major factor leading to the disorder. The theory resembles self psychology (Kohut 1971) in its assumption that children need parents to buffer their emotional distress and only learn to accomplish this task for themselves when they internalize their relationship with a caring parent. It also resembles the ideas of Winnicott (1964), who described the maternal function for the child as a "holding environment." A cognitive-behavioral theory (Linehan, 1993; Linehan and Koerner 1993) takes a similar view of parental failure in the childhood of the individual who goes on to develop BPD and describes problems in parenting as an "invalidating environment."

There also have been suggestions that the parents of borderline patients have abnormalities in their other basic task, the encouragement of autonomy and independence. Overprotection of children was described clinically in some detail by Levy (1943). Borderline patients seem to have trouble achieving autonomy, but it is not clear whether this is due to a deficit or to parental interference. A well-known psychoanalytic theory (Masterson and Rinsley 1975) suggested that a mother with BPD could influence her child to develop the same disorder if she were to selectively provide positive reinforcement for responses that maintain a mother-child symbiosis while negatively responding to behaviors that reflect individuation.

Some theorists have suggested that there could be more than one family pattern leading to BPD. Feldman and Guttman (1984) theorized that there could be two kinds of parental disturbances leading to BPD. One type involves emotionally unresponsive parents who do not recognize the affective states of their children and therefore cannot help them with emotional regulation—essentially the same hypothesis as that developed by Linehan. A second type involves one of the parents having BPD and his or her negative input to the child being unbuffered by the interventions of a second parent. This second group would be a subtype in which there is direct transmission of the condition through social learning. Such a group would have to be in the minority, because most borderline patients do not have parents with BPD (Links et al. 1988a).

Several reports based on interview data have suggested that parental bonding is abnormal in borderline patients (Frank and Paris 1981; Soloff and Millward 1983a). Researchers have also made use of a self-report instrument, the Parental Bonding Index (PBI; Parker 1983), which is specifically designed to measure adult perceptions of parental behavior during childhood. This useful tool assesses the quality of parenting through the two key dimensions of neglect and overprotection. In a recent review, Parker et al. (1992) concluded that these experiences are more related to adult social bonds in general than to intimate relationships, and that deficiencies in parenting short of gross deprivation appear capable of modification by subsequent experiences. Nevertheless, Parker has shown that psychiatric patients, most particularly those with depression, remember abnormalities in their bonding with their parents. There is also evidence that such experiences are reported more frequently in the impulsive cluster than in other personality disorders (Paris et al. 1991). It is possible that problems in parental bonding are among the multiple risk factors for BPD.

Five studies have found abnormal scores on the PBI in borderline patients (Byrne et al. 1990; R. L. Goldberg et al. 1985; Paris and Frank

1989; Torgersen and Alnæs 1992; Zweig-Frank and Paris 1991). In all of these reports, BPD patients described both neglectful and overprotective responses from their parents during childhood. The finding that parents were not only neglectful but also overprotective corresponds to what Parker (1983) has called "affectionless control." This style of parenting has been found by Parker to be particularly associated with depression in adult patients, and, in fact, the PBI scores in BPD are similar to those found in depressed patients (Parker 1983). The finding that neglectful parenting is associated with BPD has also been confirmed using structured interviews (J. C. Perry 1991). The "overprotection" scale of the PBI could be better described as measuring intrusive control, and this additional dimension could function to prevent neglected children from finding other, more protective relationships. In a recent prospective study of children followed into adulthood, only a combination of maternal overprotection and inconsistency was predictive of BPD (Bezirganian et al. 1993).

It is also of interest that the reports from borderline patients of neglect and intrusive control applied to both their parents, not just to their mothers. These results have been used to support a theory of "biparental failure" as a psychological risk factor for BPD (Frank and Paris 1981; Paris and Zweig-Frank 1993). This hypothesis proposes that when there are difficulties in bonding with both parents, the individual cannot compensate for a bad relationship with one parent by a better relationship with the other parent. There is an interesting parallel between what borderline patients report about parental bonding and their interpersonal behavior as adults, in that BPD patients show "oscillations in attachment," a pattern in which they swing from feeling empty and abandoned to being engulfed in relationships (Melges and Swartz 1989).

Although parental neglect is a risk factor for BPD, it does not appear to be specific to the disorder. As we saw in the studies of separation or loss, the specificity of psychological risk factors to BPD depends on the nature of the control group. In the studies of parental bonding cited above, borderline patients were compared either with mixed samples of outpatients or with depressed patients. In our study of psychological risk factors in female borderline patients (Paris et al. 1994a), we compared PBI scores in our BPD group with those from our control group, who had personality disorders other than BPD. We found that only one of the four scales, maternal affection, was significantly lower in the BPD group, while the other three showed no significant differences. Although this finding suggests that female borderline patients experienced more maternal neglect, the difference between the groups was small.

The pattern of scores in the male subjects in our study was somewhat different in that the borderline patients only reported higher levels of control from their fathers, although, again, there was no large difference between the BPD and non-BPD groups (Paris et al. 1994b). Nonetheless, in combination with the findings of physical abuse from fathers, as well as of frequent separation or loss (mostly of fathers), the findings for males point to an important contribution from paternal factors. Our findings were somewhat similar to the risk factors for ASPD, which are characterized by strong paternal psychopathology (L. N. Robins 1966).

When the mean scores for all our patient groups were compared with the means from normal community samples, subjects with BPD, as well as those with any type of personality disorder, reported abnormal parental bonding on all the scales of the PBI. Problems in parental bonding seem not to be specifically related to any diagnostic category, but are a general risk factor for many forms of psychopathology (Parker 1983). It is possible that there are important qualitative aspects of parent-child relationships that go beyond the broad dimensions of neglect and overprotection and are not picked up by current instruments.

In summary, there are a number of psychological risk factors for BPD, but none is quite specific to the disorder. The specificity for BPD may lie elsewhere. But before considering other possibilities, we will first examine interactions between the psychological risk factors that have been discussed in this chapter.

Multivariate Findings on the Psychological Risk Factors for Borderline Personality Disorder

All of the risk factors discussed so far have been considered more or less in isolation. But risk factors usually coexist in the same individuals.

Multivariate studies can help to determine whether psychological factors have effects independent of each other or whether the presence of one of these factors could account for the others.

In our study of female borderline patients (Paris et al. 1994a), we examined the relative contributions of trauma, neglect, and loss in the same patients to the development of BPD, using a group of control subjects with personality disorders other than BPD. As already discussed, the univariate findings were that sexual and physical abuse, as well as decreased maternal affection, were more common in the BPD group. In the multivariate analysis, only childhood sexual abuse remained significant, indicating that it has an association with BPD that is over and above its correlation with the other factors. Physical abuse and maternal affection were no longer significant, reflecting their intercorrelations with sexual abuse. Neither separation or loss nor any of the other PBI scores discriminated between the groups. These multivariate results show that the effects of childhood sexual abuse are not dependent on their association with problems in parental bonding. The results were similar in the male sample (Paris et al. 1994b), with sexual abuse and separation or loss being the two variables that differentiated BPD from other personality disorders.

There have been two other studies that parallel ours in examining psychological risk factors multivariately. In the first (Zanarini et al. 1993), the two variables that were significant were childhood sexual abuse and an absence of maternal affection. In the second (Links and van Reekum 1993), childhood sexual abuse made an independent contribution to diagnosis beyond that of physical abuse, early separation, or a measure of parental impairment.

These multivariate results suggest that the traumatic effects of sexual abuse are at least partly independent of coexisting risk factors. This independent effect points to some etiological significance for childhood sexual abuse in BPD. But these results do not necessarily mean that sexual abuse is the most important psychological risk factor for most cases of BPD. The analysis of the parameters of childhood sexual abuse suggests that this relationship is most important for a subgroup of borderline patients who had experienced more severe trauma during childhood. The degree of trauma reported by most of the borderline patients did not account for the severity of their psychopathology, nor was childhood sexual abuse specific enough to account for why some patients with this risk factor developed BPD, while others developed a personality disorder other than BPD.

Summary

The development of borderline psychopathology is not readily accounted for by any single psychological risk factor or even by groups of risk factors. There are probably multiple pathways to BPD. Histories of trauma play an important role in a subgroup of patients, while other psychological risk factors could be just as important in other cases.

J. C. Perry (1991), reporting on data from the Herman et al. (1989) study, found that childhood experiences account for about a third of the variance in borderline symptomatology, leaving two-thirds to be explained in other ways. The explanation for the lack of specificity of the psychological risk factors to BPD may not lie with childhood experience at all. It may be that psychological factors can lead to BPD only in the presence of nonpsychological risk factors.

The specific factors for BPD could be underlying personality traits. Trauma, neglect, or loss would have to interact with specific underlying personality traits to produce borderline psychopathology. In the absence of these traits, the same experiences might still produce a personality disorder, but of another category. Psychological factors would be the triggers that unleash borderline psychopathology, but not its only cause.

This interaction of the various risk factors for BPD will be discussed in more detail in Chapter 6. Before doing so, we will examine the least studied of these factors, those deriving from the social environment.

5

Social Risk Factors

O f all the elements in the biopsychosocial model, the social factors in psychiatry are the most difficult to examine empirically. We will therefore discuss how these risk factors can be studied in mental disorders in general, and then consider what research strategies could be used to determine their role in the personality disorders and specifically borderline personality disorder.

Social Risk Factors in Mental Disorders

There is no simple causal relationship between social risk and individual psychopathology. Rather, as with biological and psychological variables, social stressors can be associated with the development of specific disorders only in interaction with other risk factors. Social risk factors need not cause mental disorders in their own right, but could act by significantly lowering thresholds for psychopathology.

The general method for examining social risk factors in the major psychiatric disorders is epidemiological research. If the basic prevalence of a mental disorder is known, then we can determine if there are important variations under different social conditions. If there is variability in prevalence, it is reasonable to look for social forces that could account for it. There are a number of specific epidemiological research strategies that could be used to determine if social risk factors play a role in the etiology of a mental disorder. One strategy is to determine if the disorder has a different prevalence in different social classes. A second is to ascertain if the disorder has shown a change in prevalence over time that cannot be explained by other factors. A third strategy is to determine if a disorder shows marked differences in prevalence across cultures.

Many mental disorders are more prevalent in the lower socioeconomic classes (Dohrenwend et al. 1980). Is the link between social class and mental disorder the result of "selection and drift" (i.e., the downward social movement due to the effects of a mental disorder on social functioning), or does the association reflect causation? In a disorder such as schizophrenia, where prevalence does vary with social class, the difference is most likely due to drift (Eaton 1986; Gottesman 1991). But the stronger the psychosocial component in the development of a disorder, the more likely it is that pathological factors associated with lower socioeconomic status could themselves be etiological. However, because epidemiological findings make it difficult to establish the direction of causality, one must draw on other sources of evidence to come to a conclusion.

One phenomenon that most strongly suggests that social risk factors are involved in the etiology of a mental disorder is when there are rapid changes in prevalence over time. This procedure involves the examination of cohort differences (i.e., rates in groups who develop mental disorders at different points of history). The stronger the biological factors in a disorder, the more one would expect its prevalence to be stable. In disorders for which there are stronger psychological and social risk factors, changes in the social environment could lower the threshold for overt psychopathology. For example, dramatic increases in depression, substance abuse, and antisocial personality disorder (ASPD) (L. N. Robins and Regier 1991), as well as in the youth suicide rate over the last few decades (Sudak et al. 1984), demand some explanation involving social change.

Another test of the effect of social forces on psychopathology is cross-cultural comparisons. If a mental disorder is more frequent in one culture, or entirely confined to that society ("culture-bound"), this presents a powerful argument for social factors in etiology. One example is the wide variation in the prevalence of alcoholism across societies

(H. B. M. Murphy 1982). There are strikingly variant levels of alcoholism in different societies, which cannot be entirely attributed to differences in genetic susceptibility to alcohol, but also reflect variable social attitudes toward alcohol intake. A particularly interesting example of culture-bound syndromes is the eating disorders. These conditions are very rare in the Third World, but have attained epidemic status in developing countries (Gordon 1990). The effect of social factors on prevalence is demonstrated by the fact that eating disorders are very rare in the traditional societies from which immigrants are drawn, but show dramatic increases among the children of immigrants who move to modernized societies (DiNicola 1990). The most likely explanation is that these disorders are sensitive to cultural changes and to specific attitudes toward body shape in developed countries (Gordon 1990).

Social Risk Factors in Personality Disorders

Research Strategies

Research on social factors in the personality disorders requires specific epidemiological studies that could indicate whether personality disorders show differences in prevalence across social class, cohort, or culture. Such investigations have thus far been hampered by problems with the reliability of the diagnoses on Axis II (J. C. Perry 1992). The only personality disorder that has been systematically studied epidemiologically is the one that is also the best defined: the antisocial category. The clear-cut behavioral criteria for ASPD made it the only Axis II disorder included in the Epidemiological Catchment Area (ECA) study (L. N. Robins and Regier 1991; L. N. Robins et al. 1984).

Impulsive personality disorders, such as ASPD and BPD, are of particular interest for the social psychiatrist. First, the more observable the behavioral pathology, the more practical is epidemiological research. Second, as will be discussed later, impulsivity may be particularly sensitive to social structure. Impulsive personality disorders are also conditions of youth and have been shown to "burn out" in longitudinal follow-up studies (see Chapter 7). These disorders could therefore be useful markers for those social risk factors that have a particular impact on the young.

The first step in determining the role of social factors in the impulsive personality disorders is to establish the baseline prevalence of these disorders in the community. For this purpose instruments would have to be developed that could reliably assess the diagnostic criteria in community samples. If the prevalence of any disorder could then be shown to vary with social conditions, there would be reason to look for sociocultural factors in its etiology. Another research strategy is to study the prevalence of the personality disorders indirectly by examining the prevalence of some of their characteristic symptoms. If individual symptoms are increasing, then the disorder as a whole might be increasing in prevalence.

Social Risk Factors in Borderline Personality Disorder

Prevalence and Social Class Distribution

There are prevalence data for two of the personality disorders in the impulsive cluster. In the ECA study (L. N. Robins and Regier 1991), the 1-year prevalence of ASPD was estimated at 1.2% and the lifetime prevalence at 2.6%. There was also evidence that ASPD is on the increase in recent cohorts, based on the findings that younger people had higher rates of the disorder and that the lifetime prevalence was lower in older people.

As mentioned in an earlier chapter, there have been three estimates of the prevalence of BPD (Reich et al. 1989; Ross 1991; Swartz et al. 1990). The methods used involved either interview or questionnaire data. All three studies indicated that the disorder affects between 1% and 2% of the population, a rate that is similar to the prevalence of ASPD. The frequency of impulsive personality disorders in the population could therefore be as high as for schizophrenia. There may be many more patients with BPD than we see in our clinics.

We need to determine more precisely the community prevalence of

BPD in studies designed specifically for this purpose. Once we have done so, we can apply the research strategies discussed above to search for evidence of social influences on this prevalence. The first method involves looking for effects of social class. Swartz et al. (1990) found a trend in the direction of an association of BPD with lower educational levels, and a number of studies of personality disorders in general have shown associations with lower socioeconomic levels (Dohrenwend et al. 1980). The direction of causality is a problem, because severe personality disorders that arise early in life will interfere with education and social competence. In a clinical sample of borderline patients followed by Paris et al. (1987), more than half the cases fell in the lower socioeconomic levels because so many of these individuals failed to complete high school and did not resume their education.

We next review the results of studies that raise the possibility that there has been a recent increase in the prevalence of BPD, an increase that might be accounted for by social change.

Is the Prevalence of Borderline Personality Disorder Increasing?

Although there is no direct epidemiological evidence concerning changes in the prevalence of BPD over time, we will review indirect evidence from studies of the symptoms associated with BPD.

Although not pathognomonic of BPD, no single symptom is as suggestive of borderline pathology as repeated parasuicide (Zanarini et al. 1990b). Parasuicidal behavior has similar demographic characteristics to BPD in that it is concentrated in young females (Maris 1981). Weissman (1974) found that there had been a dramatic increase in parasuicide in young women since the 1960s, a study that should be repeated in cohorts from recent decades. It is possible that this increase reflects changes in the prevalence of BPD.

Another indirect indicator of the prevalence of BPD could be the increase in the youth suicide rate, which has tripled over the last 25 years (Sudak et al. 1984). Although this increase has occurred in males and not females, BPD could account for some of these cases, because nearly 10% of borderline patients complete suicide, in most cases while the patients are still young (Paris et al. 1989; Stone 1990). There have been four studies of youth suicide in which psychological autopsies have been carried out (Lesage et al., in press; Marttunen et al. 1991; Rich and Runeson 1992; Runeson and Beskow 1991). The psychological autopsy method, which involves obtaining information from relatives or friends, can reconstruct DSM-III-R (American Psychiatric Association 1987) Axis I and II diagnoses for individuals who complete suicide. In all four of these investigations, about one-third of the suicides were retrospectively diagnosed as being associated with BPD.

Substance abuse in the young could be another marker for BPD. Over the last 25 years the prevalence of substance abuse (Millman 1986; L. N. Robins and Regier 1991) and alcoholism (Cloninger et al. 1989; L. N. Robins and Regier 1991) has risen markedly among young people. The San Diego Suicide Study (Rich et al. 1988) also showed a strong association between youth suicide and serious substance abuse. Finally, the increase in ASPD (Robins and Regier 1991) is relevant to our discussion in that ASPD can overlap with BPD (see Chapter 2).

These findings all show that the symptoms of BPD are becoming more prevalent, and therefore suggest that the prevalence of BPD itself could be increasing. The increases in parasuicides among women, in suicide among young men, in substance abuse, and in ASPD are robust findings.

In summary, there is converging evidence of increasing prevalence for several forms of impulsivity over brief periods of time. The most probable hypothesis that could account for these dramatic shifts in behavioral symptomatology over short time periods is that the social risk factors for all of these behaviors have changed.

Cultural Factors

One of the strongest lines of evidence that would support a role for social factors in BPD would be if prevalence varies widely in different societies. We do not have firm data at present to answer this question. An ongoing study by Loranger et al. (1991) has determined that all of the Axis II disorders are diagnosable in a number of psychiatric centers around the world. However, we do not know if these clinical samples are in any way representative of nonclinical populations. Moreover, the sites for the study in the Third World were psychiatric hospitals in large urban centers. Cities in developing countries are characterized by the breakdown of traditional values under rapid acculturation and may, in fact, be settings in which there is a particularly high risk for personality disorders.

Examining specific impulsive symptoms, a number of clinical reports suggest that parasuicide, as well as youth suicide and substance abuse, has become a widespread phenomenon in many Third World countries (Paris 1991). These symptoms have been reported most frequently in urban centers and may or may not be associated with the wider range of phenomena seen in BPD.

The Third World, in which social change is particularly rapid, could be a laboratory test for the role of social factors in psychopathology. BPD should be quite rare in traditional societies. Such societies are becoming increasingly rare and are most likely to be found in rural areas. Traditional societies are characterized by intergenerational continuity in social norms and roles and by a slow rate of social change (Inkeles and Smith 1974). It will be hypothesized below that rapid social change creates conditions that are risk factors for psychopathology in general and, in particular, for disorders characterized by impulsivity. These conditions characterize contemporary urban life in developing countries.

In summary, the evidence for the role of social risk factors in BPD is indirect but suggestive. We will now consider in more detail what might be the mechanisms for these hypothesized effects.

Mechanisms for the Influence of Social Factors

There are three mechanisms by which social factors could play a role in the development of borderline psychopathology: 1) by influencing the personality dimensions that underlie the disorder (culture can shape the structure of personality by positively reinforcing some traits and negatively reinforcing others); 2) by influencing family structure and function; and 3) by interfering with the development of social roles. The concept that social environment influences personality structure was first developed by cultural anthropologists (Benedict 1961). Although the broadest personality traits are universal and do not seem to be culture-bound, there have been significant cross-national differences described for personality dimensions (Eysenck 1990). The frequency of narrowly defined traits could vary more widely from one society to another.

Influence of Social Factors on Personality Dimensions

The precise mechanism by which social factors shape enduring personality traits is unclear. At one time it was hypothesized that child-rearing practices in different cultures create modal personality types (Erikson 1950). This view seems oversimplified, because individuals in any culture have wide variations in personality. However, although the broader dimensions of personality can be found in all societies, there are significant differences on some traits (Eysenck 1982). Social value structures reward some behaviors more than others, thereby either amplifying or damping individual traits. It is possible that some personality traits are more susceptible to social influence than others. The personality dimensions that seem to underlie BPD, because they involve unstable aspects of personality, could be especially likely to be shaped by sociocultural influences. It will be the argument of this chapter that both impulsivity and affective instability are contained by one set of social factors and amplified by another set.

Influence of the Social Environment on Family Structure and Function

As reviewed in the previous chapter, there are a number of family experiences that increase the risk for borderline pathology. If social factors increase the frequency of family dysfunction, there would be a greater overall risk for BPD. Any breakdown in the social environment, such as unemployment (Eaton 1986) or the unavailability of supports from the larger community (Leighton et al. 1963), tends to increase the prevalence of mental disorders. Some of the effects of these risk factors could be due to their tendency to compromise the quality of family life and parenting. If we review the psychological risk factors discussed in the previous chapter, all of them—trauma, separation, and abnormal parenting—could be on the increase as a result of social changes. We know that nuclear families now dissolve more frequently due to separation and divorce, and it is a researchable question as to whether there have been cohort increases in the exposure of children to trauma or abnormal parenting.

Alternatively, social influences could be protective factors against psychopathology. Not all important relationships take place inside the family. The larger society can also offer alternative attachments that buffer the effects of family pathology. Extrafamilial relationships have been shown to have an important effect on personality development (Rutter and Rutter 1993). As was noted in Chapter 3, the most important nongenetic effect on personality traits comes from the unshared environment, which includes experiences outside family life. Studies of resilient children (Kauffman et al. 1979) show that relationships outside the family can be protective against even the most severe parental psychopathology. Therefore, societies that provide such relationships and make available readily accessible roles for young adults offer protection against the effects of pathology inside the family.

On the other hand, one of the social risk factors for personality disorders in modern society may be that families are smaller and more isolated from the larger community (Westen 1985). Therefore, children are less likely to receive extrafamilial buffering for family pathology.

Influence of Social Factors on the Development of Social Roles

Difficulty in establishing social roles depends not simply on the availability of jobs or marital partners, but on the requirement that young people make their own choices and obtain roles entirely through their own efforts. For those with impulsive and affectively unstable traits and with serious family pathology, these expectations may be particularly difficult to meet.

If the particular category of personality disorder that develops in an individual is determined by preexisting personality traits, then the social factors in the personality disorders need not be specific to any diagnosis. However, it remains possible that there are social risk factors that, like the psychological risk factors discussed in the previous chapter, could have a particular relationship to impulsivity. A hypothesis about the nature of these factors is explored in the next section. We then re-examine the interface between society and the family in light of this construct.

Social Disintegration

Social Disintegration as a Risk Factor for Impulsive Personality Disorders

In a classic study of social factors in mental disorders, the Stirling County study, Leighton et al. (1963) compared two Nova Scotia communities that differed on measures of a construct termed "social integration." The theoretical principles used in the Stirling County study resemble the work of Durkheim (1897/1951), which accounted for variations in the suicide rate in several European societies over time by a construct of "anomie" (i.e., normlessness). The continuum between social integration and social disintegration was measured by an index that was an amalgam of factors, such as broken homes, absence of social associations, weak leadership, few patterns of recreation, frequent crime, poverty, cultural confusion, secularization, migration, and social change. The main finding of the Stirling County study was that there was significantly more psychopathology in the more disintegrated of the two communities. The authors hypothesized that sociocultural disintegration fosters psychiatric disorders by jeopardizing physical security, by being more permissive in the expression of sexual and aggressive impulses, by interfering with loving relationships and economic success, and by interfering with finding a place in society, in a group, or in a moral order. This theory predicts that in societies that are more integrated (i.e., those with clear norms), individuals would be protected from psychopathology, whereas in societies characterized by social disintegration, psychopathology would be more likely. Although the Stirling County study was not entirely rigorous in its research methods, its concepts remain a landmark in social psychiatry and are quite relevant to contemporary phenomena.

The construct of social disintegration is an organizing principle that could help explain the social factors in mental disorders in general and in personality disorders in particular. It is also possible that social disintegration has a particular relation to impulsive personality disorders. As will be discussed, some of the most dramatic changes seen under conditions of social disintegration are substance abuse and youth suicide. The breakdown of social structures leads to a failure of social buffering. Those persons who are already vulnerable to impulsivity because of their personality traits and negative family experiences will have more difficulty obtaining supports and structures from outside the family. This hypothesis could be used to help account for the recent increase in all forms of impulsive behavior documented by epidemiological research. Increases in impulsivity are readily measurable, but they could be accompanied by less evident increases in affective instability. For example, Linehan (1993) has proposed that the relative absence of secure attachments in contemporary society increases emotional dysregulation.

Social disintegration is not a static concept. It is usually associated with the breakdown of normative structures in a society under conditions of social change. We now examine the question of whether rapid social change is itself a risk factor for impulsive personality disorders.

Social Disintegration and Rapid Social Change

Changes in the prevalence of impulsive behavior have been shown to be particularly striking under conditions of rapid social change. For example, cross-cultural studies indicate that the recent increase in suicide among the young is most apparent in several societies that have undergone particularly rapid acculturation (Jilek-Aall 1988). These findings have been striking among native populations in both North America (Jilek-Aall 1988) and Greenland (Thorslund 1990). In each case a stable traditional society was overrun by modernization, losing its historical way of life and its values. The young were particularly affected because they were unable to find social roles under new conditions.

In the past, these traditional societies had mechanisms to mimimize impulsivity and affective instability. Traditional societies offer stable social roles for their members, which are established by the community and not the individual (Westen 1985). They offer a greater level of dependence and do not encourage as much individuality as does modern society. One would therefore expect that any personality disorders in such societies would not be likely to be borderline. It is when traditional values break down that impulsive phenomena may be more likely to emerge.

A number of sociologists and contemporary historians have proposed that there has also been a breakdown of social norms in contemporary North American society (Lasch 1979a). In understanding the special vulnerability of youth to anomie, it is useful to consider Erikson's (1950) theory of adult development that describes the primary developmental task of youth: identity formation. The social expectation to form a personal identity requires a high level of individuation and autonomy. Individuals who require stronger attachment bonds may have more difficulty in establishing their independence and their goals in life.

In fact, the idea that each generation must forge its own identity is relatively new in terms of social history. In traditional societies, psychosocial roles are not chosen, but determined by the family and community. The necessity of finding one's own role is a major stressor in its own right, and young people need help from their families to make such decisions.

However, as has been noted by many observers (Lasch 1979b), the family itself is under siege in modern society. Geographical and social mobility has uprooted families from the larger community. Rapid social change seems to interfere with the transmission of values from parents to children. Although the precise effects of the recent divorce epidemic are still unclear, clinical evidence strongly suggests that children of divorce are more likely to founder during young adulthood for lack of parental guidance (Wallerstein 1989). Lasch's (1979a) description of contemporary society as "narcissistic" may not be far off the mark, considering the extent to which individualism as a value has replaced loyalty to the group (Westen 1985). Our radically individualistic society could well be characterized as disintegrated or anomic. It certainly could be defective in providing a sense of meaning and belonging for its young.

This analysis of the effects of modernization should not be mistaken for simple nostalgia (Lasch 1991). There are many benefits for the individual in modern society (Taylor 1992). Traditional societies have their own problems, and there is no reason to believe that the total weight of mental disorder is greater in contemporary civilization. It is the form of distress that is influenced by social forces. Modern society demands a higher level of individuation from its members, and there are those who will not be able to cope with such an expectation.

A high level of social demand would function as a kind of selection pressure. Some would benefit, and the effects would be neutral for the majority, but in a vulnerable minority they would lead to psychopathology. We would therefore expect to see more disorders characterized by impulsivity in societies that are undergoing rapid social change.

Social Disintegration and Family Structure

The effects of social disintegration operate at the interface between society and the family. Social norms and structures are transmitted to the individual through the nuclear family. Family structures mirror cultural values. H. B. M. Murphy (1982) has reviewed evidence that psychiatric patients in traditional societies tend to present with less impulsive behavior and more classical neurotic symptomatology. This difference could be accounted for by the containing interpersonal forces in traditional families that require repression of conflict. In contrast, the centrifugal forces in modern families could make acting out of conflict more likely (Lewis et al. 1976).

Because social forces are a factor in the cohesion and structure of families, they influence levels of family dysfunction. The findings discussed in Chapter 4 concerning psychological risk factors suggest that patients who later develop impulsive personality disorders have families that are structurally abnormal. Families with abuse and trauma are characterized by inconsistent and confused boundaries. Other family structures may fail to provide the basic levels of parental care needed to modulate dysphoric affects and to encourage the development of autonomy needed to individuate and deal with the wider world. The ability of the family to carry out its functions depends in part on social values as well as on supports from the extended family and the larger community.

Under socially integrated conditions, social structures tend to be protective against family dysfunction. These structures include the availability of alternative models for young people outside of their families, and the opportunity to find attachments in the larger community. In traditional societies, these alternatives are stable and readily accessible. Because in traditional societies adult occupational and marital roles are provided for young people rather than chosen, young people do not have to separate from their parents to the same degree as in modern families in order to forge their own psychosocial identity, and adolescence, the usual trigger for the onset of BPD, is less stressful.

In contrast, under socially disintegrated conditions, the pathology that leads to impulsive personality disorders is reinforced. Family dysfunction is more likely, and alternative sources of attachment are less available. Rapid social change may be particularly stressful for young persons who lack the inner strength and family support to develop their own identity. Moreover, adolescents are exposed to socially pathological alternatives such as substance abuse, promiscuity, and criminal activity. Most do not succumb to these temptations, because they have sufficient family support and lack impulsive predispositions. But those who are vulnerable are not protected.

Social Disintegration and Borderline Personality Disorder

The hypothesis of this chapter is that social integration is a protective factor against BPD and that social disintegration is a risk factor for BPD. These effects can be better understood by considering the core dimensions of BPD. Impulsive personality traits could be associated with sociocultural conditions in which high levels of autonomy are expected from the young at the same time that the level of social supports is decreased. Impulsivity also increases when social containment for deviant behavior decreases. Societies can either specifically proscribe characteristically "borderline" behaviors such as self-mutilation, recurrent parasuicide, and substance abuse, or create an unstructured and permissive environment in which these behaviors are more likely to occur. It is well known that rates for substance abuse vary quite widely depending on social sanctions (H. B. M. Murphy 1982). In more integrated societies, certain behaviors are not tolerated, and the distress that these behaviors communicate is either repressed or rechanneled.

As suggested by Linehan (1993), high social demand and decreased availability of attachment could also increase affective instability. In an integrated social environment, inner distress created by biological vulnerability, traumatic experiences, and dysfunctional families can be buffered by the presence of social structures that contain and modulate dysphoria. Social disintegration fosters dysphoria by offering fewer buffering and comforting structures for distress through community membership. The dimensions of impulsivity and affective instability then become mutually reinforcing. Whereas integrated societies encourage repression rather than the acting out of conflicts, less integrated social environments fail to contain dysphoria, so that those individuals with impulsive traits are more likely to act on their impulses.

The other features of BPD, such as identity diffusion, would not arise in societies that do not expect each generation to create its own identity de novo. Finally, chaotic relationships are only likely when young people are left entirely on their own to choose intimate relationships. In societies where family and community play an active role in determining object choice, the loss of freedom is balanced by an absence of unstable and rapidly disintegrating attachments.

The most prominent theorist of the social risk factors for BPD has been Millon (1987, 1993). In the context of a social learning theory of the development of BPD, Millon suggests that the anomie that characterizes contemporary society is having a particular effect on youth and is increasing the risk for borderline psychopathology. He hypothesizes that rapid social change is a risk factor for BPD in that it interferes with intergenerational transmission of values and reduces the influence of the extended family and social community.

Some Tests for the Role of Social Factors in Borderline Personality Disorder

How could these hypotheses be tested? Although social factors in mental disorders are difficult to measure, the strategies suggested earlier in this chapter could be used to provide indirect evidence for the role of social factors as risk factors for BPD. Applying the first strategy, the prevalence of BPD and its symptoms could be examined in different social environments that vary in their levels of social integration. Applying the second strategy, we could also look for cohort changes over time that are associated with changes in social integration. Applying the third strategy, we could look for cross-cultural differences in the prevalence of BPD that are associated with differences in social integration.

These tests could be carried out either in different social environments in North American society or in the rapidly urbanizing cities of the Third World, some of which demonstrate dramatic social disintegration. Studying BPD in the Third World could be instructive if there are differences between modernized and traditional settings in the same society that could help one isolate social disintegration as an etiological factor.

One setting in Western society that might also provide a useful test as to whether breakdown in the intergenerational transmission of values is associated with impulsivity would be immigrant families. Immigrant values about the separation of children from their parents tend to differ from the North American mainstream (DiNicola 1985). Although family theorists tend to see immigrant families as enmeshed (Minuchin 1974), these families could also be seen as firmly bonded (McGoldrick et al. 1982). Such families tend to tolerate lower levels of deviation and aggressivity and provide more secure attachments, even if autonomy is reduced. Beavers' (1977) theory of family structure predicts that psychopathology in the young depends on whether families are "centripetal" or "centrifugal," with the latter type leading to more behavioral pathology. There are two possible scenarios following from these theoretical considerations that could affect outcome in the children of immigrant families. Well-functioning immigrant families could have a centripetal structure that would control impulsivity. Alternatively, the stresses of acculturation for the children of immigrants could promote identity diffusion.

Summary

The research on social factors, compared with that on biological and psychological factors, is "softer," and the conclusions suggested here require more levels of inference. However, both the overall weight of the data and the theoretical considerations presented in this chapter point to an important role for social risk factors in borderline pathology. BPD does not seem to be a universal condition that can be diagnosed in all societies or in all historical periods. The prevalence of some of its characteristic symptoms varies widely from one social context to another. It seems likely that BPD is rare in traditional and socially integrated societies and that it is becoming more common in our own society as the level of social integration is declining. The influence of social risk factors can be best understood by the impact of these factors on the core dimensions of BPD.

A number of strategies have been suggested that could be used to measure more precisely the influence of social factors on BPD. In addition to these unidimensional approaches, we need to conduct studies that examine biological, psychological, and social risk factors in the same patients. The theoretical basis for biopsychosocial research on BPD is discussed in the next chapter.

6

A Multidimensional Theory of Borderline Personality Disorder

In the last three chapters we separately considered the biological, psychological, and social risk factors for borderline personality disorder. For each of these factors there is evidence—either direct or indirect—that the factor is involved in the development of BPD. None of these factors is sufficient on its own to explain the pathway to borderline personality disorder. The present chapter proposes an integrated theory of the etiology of BPD—a biopsychosocial model that will attempt to explain how personality disorders in general, and BPD in particular, could develop. Such a model involves the cumulative and interactive effects of many risk factors. It needs to consider as well the influence of protective factors—the biological, psychological, or social influences that act to prevent the development of the disorder. One note of caution is required: because the data on the etiology of BPD are rather preliminary, the discussion is necessarily theoretical and somewhat speculative. The theory presented here should be considered as a stimulus to further research.

A Biopsychosocial Theory of Personality Traits and Personality Disorders

Before examining the pathways by which a personality disorder can develop, it is important to review the distinction presented in Chapter 2 between temperament, traits, and disorders (Rutter 1987). The relationship between these constructs is summarized in Figure 6–1. *Temperament* refers to behavioral dispositions present since birth—that is, a small number of features that characterize individual differences in responding to the environment. *Traits* refer to characteristic patterns in adults—that is, complex behavioral clusters related to cognitive, emotional, and social mechanisms. *Disorders* occur when personality

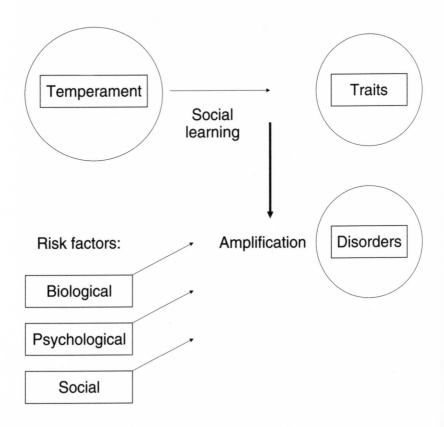

Figure 6–1. Personality: temperament, traits, and disorders.

traits interfere with occupational and/or social functioning.

Temperament reflects biological variability and therefore can be reliably observed from early childhood (Buss and Plomin 1984; Kagan et al. 1988). The broadest personality dimensions described in Chapter 2 (Buss and Plomin's emotionality, activity level, and sociability [EAS]; Eysenck's three factors) are the closest to temperament. One of the most influential theories concerning the relation of temperament to personality was developed by Chess and Thomas (1984). There are important discontinuities in temperamental factors over time (Kagan 1984). In Chess and Thomas's longitudinal study of infants, measures of temperament at birth were used to predict behavioral disturbances in childhood and adolescence. There were, in fact, few consistent relationships between infantile temperament and later functioning. By the time the subjects had reached young adulthood, the only strong predictor of later disturbance was one of the broadest measures, a "difficult" temperament (Chess and Thomas 1990). Chess and Thomas concluded that one would have to take into account interactions between temperament and parental management, which they called "goodness of fit."

These findings can be best understood if personality traits are themselves multidimensional, in that they reflect the interaction of temperament and social learning. Although traits are shaped by environmental factors, temperamental variations set limits within which this shaping can occur. The early development and persistence of character traits can be explained by these biological factors. As an example, let us consider Eysenck's dimension of extraversion-introversion. An introvert will not become an extravert, or vice versa. Rather, it is the degree of introversion or extraversion that will be open to environmental influence.

As we have seen in Chapter 3, the genetic influence on traits accounts for about 50% of the variance, leaving 50% for environmental influences. The largest portion of the environmental component in personality is unshared variance—that is, experiences unique to the individual rather than common to all children born in the same family (Tellegen et al. 1988). There are several possible explanations for the phenomenon of unshared variance. One is that there is a stronger influence on personality from experiences outside the family than has been previously postulated by developmental theories, while another possible explanation of the finding would be that parents treat different children very differently.

The psychological factors that shape personality traits could still depend in part on parental input. One hypothesis that attempts to account for this input is psychodynamic theory. This model assumes that personality is formed by family experiences early in childhood and that such experiences have a more powerful impact on personality because children are more dependent at those stages on parental responses. This theory has been difficult to support empirically, because childhood experience is highly complex and not readily open to experimental study. In fact, the hypothesis of the primacy of early experience is not consistent with evidence that the effects of even the most traumatic events in early childhood are reversible (Clarke and Clarke 1979). Moreover, theories postulating powerful effects of parental behaviors in early childhood fail to explain the dramatic differences in the personality characteristics of siblings raised in the same family (Dunn and Plomin 1990).

Some psychodynamically based theories do not assume the primacy of early experience and instead seek to explain personality development by the effects of parental influence over the entire span of childhood. In this view, traits are shaped by long-term and consistent factors in the family environment. Attachment theory is such a model, and it has been the basis of a large amount of empirical research. Main et al. (1985) have defined patterns in childhood and adult relationships that can be classified as either secure, anxious, or avoidant attachment. Attachment theory hypothesizes that these patterns are largely determined by parental behavior. When parents fail to provide secure attachment for children, anxious, avoidant, or disorganized patterns emerge. In addition, attachment styles in children tend to replicate those used by their parents. There is also some evidence that abnormal attachment is more common in the presence of an anxious temperament (Thompson et al. 1988), but, thus far, attachment theory has not considered in detail the interaction of temperament and parenting in accounting for the development of these patterns.

Another important theory of child development, emerging from the tradition of behavioral psychology, is social learning theory (Bandura

1977). Social learning theory assumes that the characteristic behavioral responses that make up personality traits are shaped by continuous reinforcement from the social environment, particularly the family. The theory also proposes that learning takes place through imitation and modeling. Social learning theory is quite consistent with observations from the family therapy literature (Minuchin 1974) in that parents may shape children's personality by defining their roles in a family structure. Because in social learning theory personality is viewed as the cumulative outcome of a large number of interactions, it would not be expected that wide changes in personality would result from single traumatic events.

Social learning theory also needs to be expanded to take into account the biological factors in personality. It could then consider temperament as a limiting factor in the shaping of behavior. The remarkable personality differences between siblings are an important example of this interaction. It seems likely that children with different temperamental dispositions respond to the same parental behaviors in quite different ways. It is noteworthy in general that parents are not predictably successful in shaping the behavior of their children. Is this simply because they are not consistent enough in their reinforcement schedules? More likely, the explanation is that parental shaping of personality is limited by temperamental factors in children.

If temperament sets limits on the behavioral repertoire of children, psychological stress would tend not to elicit new behaviors. Rather, stressful experiences would exaggerate already existing behavioral patterns. These stressors would correspond to the risk factors reviewed in earlier chapters (see Figure 6–1). Whatever the stressor, the effect would be to exaggerate and amplify the intensity of trait-linked behaviors. This theoretical principle requires empirical support. Thus far, researchers have examined the effects of acute stress on behavior, with unclear results (Lazarus and Folkman 1984). However, it could be predicted that the amplification of traits would be more likely when the stressors are chronic and enduring. This mechanism would be similar to the well-established exaggeration of personality traits seen in patients with depression (Frances and Widiger 1986).

One important stressor for any child is inadequate parental care.

The concept of "goodness of fit" (Chess and Thomas 1984) implies that effective parenting requires a high degree of flexibility and accommodation of parental strategies to the individual temperament of children. If parents apply inflexible strategies based on their own needs, their approach would be more likely to lead to amplification of unwanted traits in children. This amplification could occur whether a child was traumatized, abandoned, or neglected.

The larger social environment also plays a role in shaping personality traits. The tendency for some kinds of behavior to be more common in some cultures than in others has been found to be of sufficient clinical importance that family therapists are trained to take these differences into account (McGoldrick et al. 1982). As discussed in Chapter 5, although there are wide individual differences in personality within any culture, social factors can reinforce some traits and discourage others.

How might these various factors work interactively to determine the intensity of personality traits? Let us return to the broad personality dimension of extraversion-introversion. Extraversion reflects a strong biological predisposition. This temperamentally determined trait is entirely adaptive under normal conditions but could become unusually intense in the presence of negative environmental factors. Extraverted persons characteristically reach out to others under stress. If they experience interpersonal difficulties, they are likely to become more, not less, social. When extraverted children experience losses, trauma, or a neglectful family environment, they increase their object-seeking activities. If the stress continues, these traits may be amplified to a level that begins to be dysfunctional. For example, they may need to be a center of attention and may show protest behaviors when such attention is withdrawn. This inappropriate exaggeration of extraversion can produce negative responses. If these kinds of behaviors are used in many contexts and are associated with dysfunctional interactions, they will begin to correspond to some of the criteria for impulsive cluster personality disorders on Axis II, such as the histrionic and narcissistic types.

An introverted child, in contrast, when faced with loss, trauma, or neglect, will withdraw. Most children grow out of normal shyness (Kagan 1984); if, however, the family environment is unsupportive, introversion can become pathological, with social contacts characterized by anxiety and/or withdrawal, and an abnormal attachment pattern. Amplify this process still further and the behaviors will begin to correspond to the criteria for personality disorders of the dependent and avoidant types.

These examples demonstrate how environmental factors could determine how temperament leads to traits and how the amplification of traits could lead to disorders. Just as temperament is a limiting factor in the development of traits, traits are the limiting factor for the type of personality disorder. It is possible that when personality disorders overlap, particularly within clusters, it is because they derive from shared traits.

A Biopsychosocial Model of Borderline Personality Disorder

The theory presented in this section is similar in several respects to two others (Stone 1993a; Linehan 1993). In the model proposed by Stone (1993a), there are multiple tracks to BPD: some cases involve an etiological pathway based primarily on biological vulnerability, others develop BPD based on severe trauma without biological risk, and still others develop borderline psychopathology on the basis of an interaction between biological and psychological factors. In contrast, the model presented here assumes that all cases of BPD develop from the interaction of multiple risk factors (a neo-Kraepelinian model that adheres to a predisposition-stress theory). In the model presented by Linehan (1993), biological factors are also considered to be a necessary condition for BPD. However, Linehan hypothesizes a single dimension of genetic vulnerability, which she calls "emotional vulnerability," which resembles affective instability. In the present theory, the dimension of impulsivity is viewed as having a separate source and is not dependent on emotional dysregulation.

The model offered in this chapter for an overall biopsychosocial model for the etiology of BPD is summarized in Figure 6–2. We cannot precisely define a "borderline-prone" set of normal personality traits, but we have reviewed evidence that there are core dimensions to BPD.

These traits, impulsivity and affective instability, could be amplifications of temperamental variations. As reviewed in Chapter 2, several systems have attempted to describe these variations. Applying the EAS model of Buss and Plomin (1984), let us imagine individuals with high levels of emotionality, activity, and sociability. Those with this temperament would be emotional, active, and engaging persons who do things on the spur of the moment. Others might find them interesting, if a bit demanding.

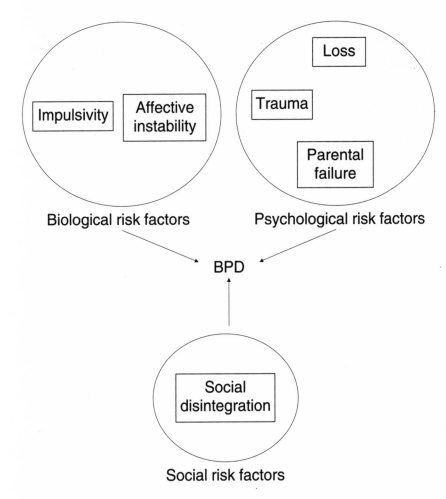

Figure 6–2. A biopsychosocial model of borderline personality disorder.

In the presence of psychological risk factors, such as trauma, loss, and parental failure, these characteristics could become amplified. Emotional reactions could become labile and dysphoric. If activity were used inappropriately to cope with dysphoria, it could become impulsive acting out. Substances, sexual activity, or chaotic interpersonal relationships could be used to damp down the dysphoria. Dysphoria and impulsive action would reinforce each other, and a feedback loop would develop. The pattern would begin to resemble BPD.

In the absence of specific underlying traits, no environmental stressor could produce this cluster of behaviors. A highly introverted person who organizes life to stay out of harm's way could develop avoidant or dependent personality disorders under stress, but never BPD. Only those persons with impulsivity and affective instability would be prone to BPD, although they could also develop a number of other disorders that share these traits, particularly those in the impulsive cluster of Axis II. It is possible that this latter group of disorders represents a continuum of psychopathology and that the more severe forms, BPD and antisocial personality disorder, only emerge when the environmental risk factors are particularly strong.

The psychological stressors that mediate amplification from trait to disorder need not be specific. The same end point could be reached by any one or combination of the most common risk factors. There would be no specific constellation in the history of the borderline patient, but rather many pathways to a final common outcome.

The future BPD patient would begin life with temperamental characteristics that are compatible with normality. If we extrapolate backward from adult personality traits, such children would be "temperamental" and more inclined toward action than reflection. But given a reasonably adequate psychosocial environment, they need never develop a personality disorder.

What, then, determines whether traits such as impulsivity or affective instability develop into BPD? There are three possibilities: 1) that the quantity of biological risk factors determines progression to disorder; 2) that environmental factors are the primary determinant of personality disorder; or 3) that the interaction of biology and environment leads to disorder. The first possibility seems unlikely, in view of the lack of evidence that personality disorders have a strong pattern of inheritance. The second possibility also seems unlikely, given the lack of a strongly specific relationship between any psychological risk factor and BPD. The preferred hypothesis in this book is the third possibility, a multidimensional and interactive model.

How would this interaction work? Again, there are several possibilities. One is that abnormal traits in children bring on negative responses from parents. Children who are impulsive and affectively labile may overlap with Chess and Thomas's (1984) category of "difficult." These children would therefore be more likely to face rejection and/or abuse if their impulsivity and emotionality make them troublesome to their families.

The other possibility is that the negative characteristics of the parents of the future borderline patient amplify personality traits in their child. The mechanisms could involve any of the psychological risk factors described in Chapter 4. Traumatic experiences in childhood, whether they occur inside or outside the family, are rooted in family dysfunction. The parents of the future borderline patient might themselves have personality disorders. They might be insensitive to the needs of their children and fail to provide an adequate holding environment. Any of these risk factors would be experienced by the child as stressful and would therefore amplify underlying personality traits.

It is noteworthy that borderline pathology does not generally begin in childhood, but in adolescence. We lack the longitudinal data that would allow us to identify what kind of children later develop BPD. There is no evidence, either, that borderline patients have clear-cut psychopathology as children or that many children with psychopathology later develop BPD. The onset of the disorder in adolescence could indicate that those who have the risk factors for BPD are less likely to be able to manage the developmental tasks of that phase.

The social environment could act either as a risk factor or as a protective factor. Even in the presence of a biological predisposition and a traumatic or inadequate family environment, a positive social environment could prevent the development of BPD by providing structures that buffer dysphoria and impulsivity. Based on this model, BPD would be less frequent in highly integrated societies where family structures are stronger and where children have alternative sources of bonding, which makes them less emotionally dependent on what happens in the nuclear family. On the other hand, in societies with higher levels of social disintegration, many adolescents would have increased difficulty with the transition to adult roles, and those who are prone to borderline pathology might begin to show the characteristic features of the disorder.

In general, it is the balance between risk factors and protective factors that would determine how likely it would be for any individual to develop BPD. The personality traits that increase the risk for BPD could be buffered by other traits that protect against BPD. Protective psychological factors could involve positive experience with secure attachment figures. Protective social factors would include those that have been established as being linked with resilience in children, such as important relationships outside the family and experiences in school (Rutter 1987).

In summary, a biopsychosocial model of BPD begins with those biological factors that could explain the specificity of the disorder. These factors are linked theoretically to temperament, but can best be measured in adults by personality traits. These traits, which are shaped by the interaction of temperament and environment, would collectively be the limiting factor that determines what type of personality disorder can develop in any individual. Psychological as well as social factors could amplify the intensity of these traits to dysfunctional levels. Each of the risk factors would be necessary but not sufficient conditions to produce any personality disorder. The sufficient conditions would be a combination of all of the risk factors.

The biopsychosocial model for the etiology of BPD offered in this chapter is heuristic but clearly provisional. It is consistent with the available evidence but lacks specific empirical support at many crucial points. In Chapter 10, a research strategy to test some of the hypotheses derived from the theory will be suggested.

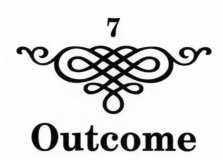

7

Outcome

I n this chapter we examine the long-term outcome of borderline patients and attempt to understand the course of borderline personality disorder in terms of its core dimensions.

Schmideberg (1959) described the course of BPD as "stably unstable," and several early follow-up studies seemed to confirm this view. When reexamined 5 years after initial presentation, most borderline patients show very little change (Carpenter et al. 1977; Pope et al. 1983; Werble 1970).

In the last decade, there have been four studies that followed patients for 15 years (McGlashan 1985, 1986; Paris et al. 1987, 1988; Plakun et al. 1985; Stone 1990), and a fifth study conducted a 10-year follow-up (Silver and Cardish 1991). All these investigators found that most borderline patients improve over the long term (Paris 1988, 1993b). These important findings are worth examining in some detail.

Long-Term Studies: Global Outcome and Suicide

The 15-year outcome studies of BPD are an example of scientific serendipity. Four groups who did not know of one another's existence undertook research, and all published their findings at about the same time. McGlashan (1985, 1986) followed a cohort admitted to Chestnut Lodge, a private psychiatric hospital near Washington, D.C. Stone

(1987, 1990, 1993b) studied a cohort from a unit established by Columbia University in New York for the long-term residential treatment of personality disorders. The present author, along with Drs. Ronald Brown and David Nowlis (Paris et al. 1987, 1988, 1989), followed patients from an urban general hospital, Jewish General Hospital in Montreal. Plakun et al. (1985, 1991) obtained data from patients who had been admitted to the Austen Riggs Center, a private psychiatric hospital in Massachusetts. The fifth, unpublished study, by Silver and Cardish (1991), is still in progress and is following patients from the inpatient ward of a general hospital, Mount Sinai in Toronto.

In all the studies, baseline diagnoses of BPD were established retrospectively from chart review using criteria from either DSM-III (American Psychiatric Association 1980) or the Diagnostic Index for Borderlines (DIB). All the researchers measured global outcome at follow-up using either the Health-Sickness Rating Scale (HSRS; Luborsky 1962) or the Global Assessment Scale (GAS; Endicott et al. 1976); in addition, a variety of scales were used to assess specific outcomes such as work, relationships, symptomatology, and further hospitalizations.

As one might expect, each study had some methodological limitations. One important issue in follow-up research is to locate as many subjects as possible from the original sample. The studies varied widely, with the McGlashan and Stone studies having the highest percentage of subjects located (over 80%), whereas both the present author's group and Plakun's succeeded in locating less than a third of their cohort. Although the three studies (McGlashan, Plakun, Paris) that carried out bias testing on the non-follow-up subjects found few differences in baseline data from the located sample, one can never be sure that the missing subjects would not have differed on the outcome measures.

In three of the studies (McGlashan, Stone, Paris), outcome was assessed largely through telephone interviews. Although McGlashan compared data obtained from face-to-face and phone interviews and found few differences, there might still be qualitative losses from using the telephone. Silver and Cardish, who have carried out only face-to-face interviews, suggest that in-depth interviewing reveals more subtle psychopathology. In one study (Stone 1990), functioning was assessed in many cases from reports by key informants, and in another (Plakun et al. 1985), the data were drawn from a self-report questionnaire.

In spite of these limitations, there was a remarkable concordance in the findings. This concordance was all the more striking since the samples were so different, and our own cohort came not from a residential or private hospital setting but from an urban general hospital. By the time they reached middle age, the majority of patients no longer had acute symptoms, and in our cohort most (75%) no longer met the diagnostic criteria for BPD. The mean global outcome scores were nearly identical among the studies, falling in the mid-60s. (An HSRS or GAF score in this range reflects mild difficulties and can be considered as within the range of normality.) In our study, when subjects were rediagnosed using the DIB, all of the subscales (dysphoria, impulsivity, disturbed relationships, and micropsychotic phenomena) showed decreased scores over time. In all of the studies, rehospitalization was uncommon after the first few years, and most patients on follow-up were working and had a social life. However, it is not clear that recovery over time in BPD is complete, because many patients were prone to further psychiatric disorders (McGlashan 1986; Silver and Cardish 1991), and about 25% continued to meet the criteria for BPD (Paris et al. 1987). But in the majority of cases, BPD remits by early middle age.

The down side of the story is the high rate of completed suicide in BPD. Both Stone and the present author's group found rates of 8% to 9%, and have learned of additional suicides since their results were published. A much lower rate of 3%, reported by McGlashan (1986), is most probably not truly representative of the borderline population, because patients admitted to Chestnut Lodge are sifted from treatment failures in general hospitals and are somewhat older than patients in the other samples, and patients likely to commit suicide may have already done so prior to being admitted for residential treatment (T. H. McGlashan, personal communication, 1991). Confirmation of the high frequency of suicide in BPD comes from two recent Norwegian studies, one reporting a suicide rate of 8% (Kjelsberg et al. 1991) and the other, 10% (Aarkrog 1993), as well as from Silver and Cardish (1991), who found that 10% of their sample had suicided after 10 years. We can therefore conclude that 1 in 10 borderline patients will go on to eventually complete suicide. This rate is similar to that found in schizophrenia

(Wilkinson 1982) and mood disorders (Guze and Robins 1970). Most of these suicides occur in the first 5 years of follow-up.

Can we predict which patients are most at risk, either for poor outcome or for suicide? Such predictors could be demographic factors such as education, measures of functional level before treatment, clinical measures such as particular symptoms or diagnostic criteria, or developmental factors such as traumatic events during childhood. McGlashan (1985) found two of the strongest predictors of good global outcome to be higher IQ and shorter length of previous hospitalization. These factors did not, however, account for a large percentage of the variance and are likely to be predictive of the outcome of many psychiatric disorders. The only clinical predictor in the McGlashan study that might be specific to BPD was affective instability, a finding confirmed in our own study. Plakun et al. had different results: using DSM-III criteria, they found that self-damaging acts and inappropriate anger were the best predictors of a poor outcome.

Several researchers have looked for a relationship between developmental factors and global outcome. The findings are suggestive but not very consistent. In our study (Paris et al. 1988), there was a correlation between an index of problems with mothers during childhood and lower outcome scores. Stone (1990) emphasized a relationship between outcome and a measure of "parental brutality," but this variable accounted for only 7% of the variance in a multiple regression. More recently, in the study reported in Chapter 4 (Paris and Zweig-Frank 1993), we found that severe childhood sexual abuse was somewhat more frequent in women with BPD who remained symptomatic when compared with a sample of the same age who had recovered, a relationship that was also found by Links et al. (1993). Both Links et al. (1993) and Zanarini et al. (1993) have found that in the follow-up of prospective cohorts, continued substance abuse is the strongest predictor of failure to recover from BPD. But none of these results is robust enough to provide clinically useful predictors of outcome.

We also lack good predictors for suicide in BPD. In part, this is unsurprising, because completed suicides are a rare event and difficult to predict, even in large samples of patients (Pokorny 1983). There have been suggestive but inconsistent findings from the long-term outcome studies. Stone (1990) found that borderline patients with substance abuse were more likely to suicide, which makes sense, because substance abuse itself carries a high risk of suicide (Flavin et al. 1990). Paris et al. (1989) found that previous attempts predicted later completion. This finding has been confirmed by a Scandinavian study (Kullgren 1988) that compared borderline patients who completed suicide after psychiatric admission to those who stayed alive. The relationship of previous attempts to completion is a general finding in suicide research (Maris et al. 1992). Because parasuicide in BPD can be seen by clinicians as only "manipulative," it is important to understand its prognostic import. However, suicide attempts by overdose should be distinguished from self-mutilation or wrist slashing, which have not been shown to have any relationship to ultimate suicide (Kroll 1993).

Because our sample differed from the others in having a wide range of socioeconomic levels, we were able to examine whether social class predicts outcome in BPD. Although education was not related to global outcome, patients with higher education were somewhat more likely to complete suicide (Paris et al. 1988). A parallel finding has been reported in schizophrenic patients by Drake et al. (1984), in whose study high social class and high expectations were associated with suicide. In some cases, suicide seems to result from the contrast between high expectations in life and a chronic, disabling mental illness. However, a report from Norway failed to replicate this relationship between social class and suicide in BPD (Kjelsberg et al. 1991).

There have been some findings that link developmental history with suicide completion in BPD. For example, Kjelsberg et al. (1991) found that borderline patients who experienced separation or loss early in life were more likely to complete suicide, a result that was also found in a recent psychological autopsy study of young male borderline individuals who had completed suicide (Lesage et al. 1993). However, in our own follow-up, we found that patients who completed suicide actually had a less traumatic childhood, reflecting our intercorrelations of suicide with higher education (Paris et al. 1988).

Prospective studies are needed to define more clearly the predictors of both long-term outcome and suicide in BPD. There have been several such cohorts established. In the Boston area, J. C. Perry (1985) followed a cohort for 7 years, and Zanarini (1993b) is now carrying out a major prospective study. The most important results thus far have come from an ongoing study in Hamilton, Ontario (Links et al. 1990a, 1993), which found that at 7-year follow-up, over a third of the cohort were already no longer diagnosable as having BPD (Links et al. 1993).

There are, nonetheless, problems with prospective research designs. In prospective studies there is inevitably attrition (i.e., the loss of subjects over time). Another problem is that borderline patients who are compliant enought to agree to be followed longitudinally could have unusual characteristics—ones that may or may not correspond to the larger universe of borderline patients seen by clinicians. Nonetheless, prospective research offers the best way to identify more clinically useful predictors of ultimate outcome in BPD.

Mechanisms of Change

Borderline personality disorder is one of a number of conditions that seem to "burn out" as patients grow older. Even the positive symptoms of schizophrenia are less apparent in late middle age (Harding et al. 1987a, 1987b). Many of the syndromes that improve with age belong to the group of "impulse spectrum disorders" (Zanarini 1993a), such as substance abuse (L. N. Robins and Regier 1991; Vaillant 1973, 1983) and antisocial personality disorder (Maddocks 1970; L. N. Robins and Regier 1991). In both of these conditions a majority of cases no longer show the behavioral manifestations of the disorder by middle age, although there is a significant mortality prior to "burnout."

The commonality with other impulsive disorders suggests one possible mechanism for change in BPD. Even in normal populations, impulsivity is associated with youth. Vaillant (1977) found that immature defenses are replaced by more mature defenses when individuals are followed over time. Bond et al. (1983) also found that defenses characterized by impulsive action decrease with age. Neuroticism is reduced from age 17 to age 30 and remains stable thereafter (Costa and Widiger 1994).

These changes in impulsivity could reflect brain maturation, such that biological risk factors, such as neurotransmitter levels, undergo change with time. The changes could also reflect social learning. In either case, it seems likely that the decrease of impulsivity with age is one of the main mechanisms of recovery in BPD.

It is not clear whether the affective instability of the borderline patient changes to the same extent as does impulsivity. Although the outcome studies show that borderline patients in middle age are less clinically depressed, Silver and Cardish (1991) suggest that "burned out" borderline patients retain an inner core of dysphoria and chaos that can be elicited by a skilled interviewer.

The core dimensions of BPD could mature from biological development or from social learning. In a report by Bardenstein and McGlashan (1989) and in our own cohort (Paris et al. 1987), it was noted that many borderline patients seemed to reduce their symptoms by restricting their relationships and "staying out of trouble." Because it is intimate relationships that so often bring on symptoms in BPD, patients can reduce their symptomatology simply by avoiding the situations they cannot handle. Sublimations, such as involvement in work, can provide satisfying substitutes for intimacy.

McGlashan's (1986) finding that the borderline patients over age 50 in his sample were doing more poorly and having trouble with alcohol abuse is a sign that recovered BPD cases may remain susceptible to breakdown as they suffer losses in later life. There is even some evidence that borderline patients can be found in geriatric populations (Sadavoy 1992). The continuing fragility of the aging formerly borderline patient could be better assessed if we had 25- and 35-year follow-up data.

Implications for Clinical Management

One important implication of outcome research for treatment is that it is difficult to assess the efficacy of therapy for a disorder marked by relapses and chronicity. It would be easy to confound naturalistic changes with treatment effects. Borderline patients tend to get better with time, either by reducing impulsivity or by learning to avoid intimacy. It is, of course, also possible that they may improve more rapidly with treatments such as psychotherapy. But only clinical trials can determine whether treatment affects course. These trials would have to follow up patients over a long-term period, because clinical experience with this population suggests that short-term improvements are often unstable. Paradoxically, however, results within 5 years would be more likely to reflect treatment effects than improvement over longer periods, when naturalistic improvement holds sway.

It is of interest that while four of the five long-term outcome studies offered residential treatment and intensive psychotherapy, our general hospital study had the same outcome results in a sample of patients who received only short-term hospitalization followed by intermittent crisis intervention. Although differences between the samples do not allow using the data to determine treatment effectiveness, the long-term effects of more intensive therapy remain to be demonstrated. Furthermore, in view of the high suicide rate among BPD patients, even among those who receive intensive therapy, we cannot claim to know how to prevent suicide in this population.

Descriptions of treatment for BPD generally suggest a long and difficult process. It is not clear whether this is because treatment takes time or because therapy is a delaying action that keeps patients alive until they improve naturalistically with time. BPD is clearly a chronic illness with formidable morbidity and mortality. Although improvement over the long term is the most common outcome, it is by no means certain. In this light, many of the principles used for the management of chronic medical conditions could be applied to BPD. There are a number of parallel conditions in medicine that improve with age. One example would be bronchial asthma, which can be a life-threatening illness early in life but gradually remits in severity over time, albeit with later relapses.

In any chronic illness, the therapeutic enterprise can best be seen as mediating, buffering, and holding, rather than being strictly curative. Patients need to be offered a range of options that will maintain them on as comfortable a level as possible until they improve. McGlashan (1993) suggests that the outcome literature supports a therapy of BPD that is intermittent, continuous, and eclectic. In other words, treatment should be adapted to the chronicity of the disorder. Treatment can be *intermittent* because we need not expect complete recovery from the disorder, and because once an alliance is formed, patients will benefit most from interventions when they are facing acute problems. Treatment needs to be *continuous* because patients are susceptible to relapse. Finally, treatment has to be *eclectic* because there is no single modality that is uniquely effective. In the next chapter we will consider all possible treatment options for BPD in the light of these principles.

8

Treatment Options

The Dimensions of Treatment for Borderline Personality Disorder

The outcome findings discussed in the previous chapter could be cause for either pessimism or optimism about treatment. On the one hand, the chronicity of BPD is humbling and raises serious questions about the effectiveness of our current therapies. On the other hand, the naturalistic improvement that occurs in BPD over time raises the possibility that if we could understand its mechanism, then we might be able to find ways to make recovery proceed more rapidly.

It would also be surprising if a disorder with a complex etiology could be treated effectively with a single therapeutic modality. Most borderline patients require multimodal treatment. The biological, psychological, and social risk factors discussed in the earlier chapters of this book could therefore help to shed light on how to treat BPD. The core dimensions of BPD could be particularly useful in identifying the mechanisms by which therapy could modify the symptoms of BPD and in defining more specific targets for our treatment strategies.

One of the primary aims of any form of treatment for borderline patients is to control impulsivity. There are a number of possible ways to achieve this goal. Biological interventions could have a direct damping effect on impulsivity by acting on those neurotransmitter systems that modulate behavioral control, or an indirect effect by acting on those neurotransmitter systems that control the dysphoria which can lead to impulsivity. Psychological interventions could combat impulsivity by reframing emotional reactions through cognitive restructuring or interpretation; by teaching, through psychoeducational measures, behavioral control; or by providing a holding environment to relieve dysphoria. Interventions that introduce structure into the social environment of patients could also reduce the frequency of impulsive actions.

The other core dimension of BPD, affective instability, could be influenced in similar ways. Pharmacological methods could be developed to decrease the sensitivity of mood to environmental changes. Psychotherapeutic measures could stabilize mood by providing a supportive relationship, as well as by helping patients to monitor their emotional responses to others. Social interventions could influence levels of environmental support that could buffer affective instability.

Thus far, the treatments that have been shown empirically to be useful in BPD seem to have their most dramatic effect in damping down the impulsive dimension of the disorder, whereas the treatments designed to control the affective instability of the borderline patient seem to be less successful. In the future we may develop treatments with greater specificity for both core dimensions.

Clinical Trials and Caveats

Therapists treating borderline patients have tended to rely on the recommendations of senior clinicians who are experienced in dealing with these difficult cases. But only controlled trials can tell us which methods of treatment are consistently effective. Therefore, in discussing the options for therapy of BPD in this chapter, the emphasis is on those interventions that have been evaluated by clinical trials. However, methodological problems, which apply to the investigation of treatment modalities for any psychiatric disorder, raise difficulties in the interpretation of these trials. It is therefore necessary to provide some caveats.

Sampling Problems

Patients who enter clinical trials are not necessarily representative of the larger population of patients with a given diagnosis. For example, the referral process to any clinic involves a process of sifting out, either of the least severe or of the most severe cases. Patients who agree to participate in clinical trials may be more compliant than those who do not. Borderline patients are in fact particularly known for their noncompliance with recommended treatment, and there are reports that they present major problems when asked to enter clinical trials (Links and Boiago 1992). Therefore, reports of successful trials must be tempered by the question of which patients agreed to participate.

Specific and Nonspecific Effects of Treatment

When clinical trials do show that treatment is effective, it is not always clear what mechanism accounts for the positive outcome. Good results could be due either to specific technical aspects of therapy or to nonspecific factors that are common to many forms of treatment. This question has arisen most particularly in assessing research findings on the outcome of psychotherapy.

There is now a large body of data which shows that psychotherapy is reasonably effective in a wide range of patients (Garfield and Bergin 1986; Smith et al. 1980). However, no particular method has been shown to work better than any other (Garfield and Bergin 1986; Luborsky et al. 1975). There is also robust evidence that the outcome of therapy is much more strongly related to characteristics of the patient than to those of the therapist (Garfield and Bergin 1986; Strupp and Hadley 1979). The most likely explanation is that the effects of psychotherapy are common to all methods and are nonspecific in relation to technique or theory. Therefore, clinical trials of psychotherapy in BPD that demonstrate a successful outcome should not necessarily be interpreted as showing that the results are due to the particular technique applied in the study.

Heterogeneity of the Borderline Personality Disorder Patient Population

Any findings about the overall effectiveness of treatment in BPD may be misleading unless differences between subpopulations of borderline patients are taken into account (Waldinger 1987). There may be subgroups based on such characteristics as symptomatology, demographics, or external competence. It is possible that these characteristics, which are independent of clinical diagnosis, could be important predictors of treatment response. Subgroups defined by such characteristics might respond differently to various combinations of psychotherapies, pharmacological agents, or behavioral training procedures.

With these caveats in mind, the major options for treatment of BPD can be considered.

Treatment Options

Option 1: Pharmacological Interventions

Borderline patients have prominent psychiatric symptoms and are often given pharmacological treatment to control these symptoms. These interventions often target a comorbid Axis I diagnosis, such as major depression. At times, the Axis II diagnosis is not even made, because it can suggest to clinicians that the patients will not respond to treatment. There are also times when pharmacotherapy in BPD reflects the frustrating nature of this disorder. Some borderline patients are treated with polypharmacy: when one medication stops working, a new one is added, until the patient is receiving four or five. An additional problem is that borderline patients can be both noncompliant and abusive in their use of medication (Waldinger and Frank 1989).

There is, however, an empirical basis for psychopharmacological treatment in BPD, and clinical trials now offer a substantial amount of data (Soloff 1990, 1993). The strongest positive effects seem to be with low-dose neuroleptics (Cowdry and Gardner 1988; S. C. Goldberg et al. 1986; Serban and Siegel 1984; Soloff et al. 1986; Teicher et al. 1989). There are two groups of symptoms in BPD that could be targeted by these drugs: impulsivity and micropsychotic phenomena. The evidence from the aforementioned studies shows that neuroleptics reduce impulsivity in borderline patients, but that the level of change, although statistically significant, is clinically marginal. Although neuroleptics curb impulsivity, they are not known to have a specific effect on the neurotransmitter systems modulating these behaviors. Low-dose neuroleptics may be effective, but patients tend to feel quite dysphoric while taking them. Moreover, in view of their side effects, and in the absence of evidence of their long-term usefulness (Cornelius et al. 1993), these agents should probably be used for a short duration, either when impulsivity is out of control or when specific treatment of micropsychoses is indicated.

It should be noted that there is no effect of psychopharmacological interventions on the interpersonal difficulties that accompany the behavioral disturbances in BPD. Psychobiological theory (Siever and Davis 1991), which postulates a specific relationship between neurotransmitter systems and personality traits, could be the basis for developing new drugs to more narrowly target trait symptomatology such as impulsivity.

The value of antidepressants in BPD is problematical. As discussed by Gunderson and Phillips (1991), the relatively weak and inconsistent response of borderline patients to tricyclics is one of the reasons for rejecting the hypothesis that BPD is a subaffective dysthymia. Soloff et al. (1986) even described cases in which amitriptyline seemed to make BPD worse. There seems to be more evidence for the usefulness of monoamine oxidase inhibitors (MAOIs). The use of tranylcypromine for control of affective instability was described many years ago by Klein (1977) in a patient population with what Klein called "hysteroid dysphoria," but who would probably have met BPD criteria. Cowdry and Gardner (1988) and Soloff (1993) have reported results with MAOIs that are statistically significant but not clinically impressive. As Soloff (1993) summarized, "Symptom change was modest at best, with residual symptoms the rule."

It is worth noting that a number of studies have shown that the presence of any personality disorder on Axis II seems to make the treatment of depression, whether by pharmacotherapy or psychotherapy, less successful (Shea et al. 1990). This is a practical reason why Axis II diagnoses should not be missed, and it suggests that a diagnosis of BPD is a good reason for caution in using antidepressants.

It is possible, however, that the specific serotonin reuptake inhibitors (SSRIs) will prove to be more effective in BPD. Given the evidence that BPD is associated with a sluggish serotonergic system (Coccaro et al. 1989), one would expect that the most effective drug for borderline patients would be an SSRI. Therefore, particular interest has been taken in assessing the efficacy of fluoxetine in BPD. There have been three open trials for its use in BPD patients (a total of 35 patients) (Cornelius et al. 1990; Markowitz et al. 1990; Norden 1989), all of which reported some improvement. Recently reported double-blind, placebo-controlled trials (Markowitz 1993) suggest that some patients improve dramatically, particularly in terms of the control of self-mutilation, but that others drop out, partly due to side effects. The follow-up data suggested to the investigators that there is a significant minority who benefit from fluoxetine but that the medication is far from universally effective. Sertraline may be more useful than fluoxetine, because it is better tolerated (Markowitz 1993).

Using any pharmacological agent in borderline patients requires taking into account the risk of overdose. Fluoxetine has an obvious advantage in BPD, because it has been shown to be relatively safe when overdoses are taken (Blackwell 1987). There has been concern about whether fluoxetine is associated with increases in suicidal ideation (Teicher et al. 1990). However, it is difficult to assess such effects in a population of patients who are already highly suicidal. Increases in suicidality are known to occur with all antidepressants, and there is no reason to believe that fluoxetine carries a more specific risk. In a survey of outpatients treated with either fluoxetine or tricyclics for depression (Fava and Rosenbaum 1991), there was no difference in suicidal complications between the two drug groups, and the effects observed were not as severe as those described by Teicher et al. in their series of six cases.

The other drugs that are used in the treatment of mood disorders and that have been tried in BPD are lithium and carbamazepine. Links et al. (1990b) found marginally positive effects for lithium, which would not seem to justify its use for borderline patients in general, although there could be a subgroup who would benefit. The theory behind trying carbamazepine was that BPD has a neurobehavioral component, possibly associated with abnormal limbic activity, that might respond to an anticonvulsant. The drug is hypothesized to have a damping effect on affective instability, but Gardner and Cowdry (1986) found it more effective against impulsive dyscontrol. Carbamazepine might offer a less toxic alternative to low-dose neuroleptics.

It is worth pointing out that benzodiazepines are generally contraindicated in BPD, in view of their disinhibiting effects on impulsivity (Stein 1992). Anxiety symptoms in BPD are probably better managed with low-dose neuroleptics.

In summary, pharmacological intervention in BPD could be indicated on a short-term basis when impulsivity is out of control. It is not clear that we have effective pharmacotherapy for the unstable mood seen in BPD. The chronic characterological problems of the borderline patient need to be approached by nonpharmacological means. We should, however, be open to the possibility that in the forthcoming years we will have drugs that are more specific to the traits underlying BPD.

Option 2: Hospitalization and Day Treatment

Borderline patients have been described as constituting 26% of inpatients in some settings (Gunderson 1984). Most frequently, admission arises from attempted or threatened suicide. There are several controversies about the value of hospital treatment for BPD patients. In the first place, although borderline patients are characterized by chronic suicidality, it has not been shown that hospitalization prevents suicide in this patient population (Paris 1993b). In the second place, when BPD patients are admitted to the hospital, it is not known whether the stay should be short-term or long-term. Finally, it is possible that hospitalization can have negative effects in borderline patients (Dawson 1988; Dawson and MacMillan 1993).

To know whether hospitalization prevents suicide in BPD, we would need randomized trials in which patients are either admitted or not admitted to the hospital after presenting with suicide attempts or threats. Such studies have not been done for obvious ethical reasons. Nevertheless, BPD patients are usually hospitalized when they seem to be acutely suicidal. Clinicians may be motivated by the fear of being held responsible for a fatality, and they may utilize the hospital to protect the patient by close observation. Problems tend to arise around discharge, which often precipitates more suicidal ideas (Silver and Rosenbluth 1993). Outcome research has shown that the highest risk for suicide does not, in fact, occur at the time of hospitalization, but later on, when the patient is more isolated and disconnected (Paris et al. 1989; Stone 1990). When borderline patients complete suicide, they usually do so after a series of failed treatments, rather than in the midst of active therapy.

If the suicidal borderline patient is hospitalized, there should be a specific treatment plan to reduce the suicide risk. If we had more specifically effective psychopharmacological interventions to offer, and if hospitalization, as with the functional psychoses, offered an opportunity to institute such treatment in a controlled environment, then there would be stronger reasons to admit BPD patients to the hospital. In the absence of such specific measures, hospitalization is a holding operation.

When hospitalization is carried out for borderline patients, it tends in most settings to be brief and to target the control of impulsive symptoms (Silver and Rosenbluth 1993). One factor influencing treatment in American hospitals is the growth of managed care, because longer stays are not generally reimbursed. There has been some controversy as to whether borderline patients should be admitted briefly, or whether they can benefit from longer hospitalizations or residential treatment. Again, there are few empirical data on which to base conclusions. The most relevant research has been a series of studies examining length of hospitalization (Glick et al. 1977), which found no correlation between outcome and length of stay in a variety of diagnostic pictures, including personality disorders. I. D. Glick (personal communication, 1991) thinks that many of the patients in this series of studies would at present be diagnosed as having BPD. Given the massive use of resources required for long-term hospitalization, the burden of proof falls on those who support the more expensive option.

Some of the characteristics of inpatient units have the potential to make BPD patients worse (Dawson 1988). It is common enough to see an escalation of impulsivity in a hospitalized patient. The problem seems to be the lack of structure, particularly in programs that are focused on emotional expression rather than activity. Such highly ambiguous, intermittently gratifying and frustrating milieus may even resemble some of the circumstances these patients report in their families of origin (Melges and Swartz 1989).

An alternative to full hospitalization, and one that is probably underutilized, is day treatment. This modality has many of the advantages claimed for admission, such as a better opportunity to build a treatment alliance or to introduce more intensive modes of therapy than can be undertaken in an outpatient setting. But it lacks the disadvantages of full hospitalization, because day treatment programs have less unstructured activities that can lead to regression. Day programs are activity oriented and use time in a highly structured way. In this environment, chronically suicidal patients can be observed and managed with less possibility of complications. Good results have been documented in a Norwegian follow-up of patients in day treatment (Friis 1993). A comparative trial of full and partial hospitalization would be needed to test the hypothesis that day programs are particularly useful in BPD.

Option 3: Psychodynamic Psychotherapy

Although many books (Adler 1985; Gunderson 1984; Kernberg 1984) have been written about psychodynamic therapy for borderline patients, it remains a controversial option. Most of the literature is based on a limited number of cases who may not be typical of borderline patients as a group (Aronson 1989) and for whom investigators did not spell out specific indications and contraindications for such therapy.

Open-ended, intensive psychodynamic psychotherapy involves seeing patients several times a week in an open-ended time frame. The method is characterized by emphasis on the uncovering of childhood experience and on interpretation of the transferences that recapitulate such experiences. There are several problems in assessing the value of this approach. In the first place, it has never been subjected to rigorous clinical trials; most of the evidence for its effectiveness is anecdotal. In the second place, even when patients do improve with intensive long-term therapy, it has never been shown that they are responding to any specific technique. In studies of patients in psychodynamic psychotherapy, when they are asked what had been most helpful in their therapy, most of them emphasized the relationship with the therapist (Strupp et al. 1969). For borderline patients in particular, the "corrective emotional experience" (Alexander and French 1946) could be the most important factor. The need of the borderline patient to have a positive experience in therapy has also been described as involving the mechanism of introjection, either of the supportive aspects of the therapy (Adler 1985) or of the therapeutic alliance (Horwitz 1974). It should also be noted that psychodynamic therapy, like any other psychotherapy, involves a great deal of "working through" (i.e., discussion of how to manage difficulties in the patient's present life experiences). It therefore contains important components that overlap with cognitive and behavioral therapies (Wachtel 1977).

Finally, it is far from clear that all therapists follow the same procedures when performing psychodynamic therapy. An advance in this respect is the development of manuals that describe treatment procedures in detail. A manual has recently been developed for one model of dynamic therapy for BPD (Kernberg et al. 1990), which will allow researchers to begin to study the method systematically (Clarkin et al. 1992).

Some authors who have been critical of the claims that have been made for psychodynamic therapy in BPD have suggested that supportive forms of treatment are more appropriate for most borderline patients. For example, Friedman (1975) has argued that intensive psychotherapy is unnecessary at best and dangerously regressive at worst. Friedman raises the question as to whether intensive therapy makes some BPD patients worse. In a review of a book (Waldinger and Gunderson 1987) describing dynamic treatment of a small number of BPD cases, Friedman (1989) concluded that "good results are of course important, but this book reminds us that we must ask at what price they are achieved and if there is a more effective, less destructive mode of achieving the same results" (p. 1337).

The danger of long-term intensive psychodynamic therapy lies in its failure to provide the structures that borderline patients need. As we have seen in Chapters 4 and 5, structure, in both the family and social environments, is a protective factor that makes BPD less likely to develop. When borderline patients are initially evaluated, they often demonstrate disorganization if the interview is inadequately structured. The more questions one asks, the more healthy the patient looks; but if one does not ask questions, the patient's pathology emerges. This phenomenon of a regressive response to an unstructured task can also be picked up by psychological testing, and in the original description by Gunderson and Singer (1975) it was even considered to be a defining characteristic for BPD. A number of studies they reviewed have shown that when borderline patients are presented with an unstructured stimulus, such as a Rorschach blot, the patients have difficulty in organizing their response cognitively and may be scored as showing quasi-psychotic thinking; whereas when they are asked to do more defined activities, such as answering questionnaires, they appear much more normal.

Classical psychoanalysis has, with some exceptions, been considered to be contraindicated for BPD. In fact, its failure to help these patients was the basis of Stern's (1938) original paper. The procedure of daily sessions on a couch, which are specifically designed to be ambiguous in order to loosen neurotic defenses, is not tolerated by most borderline patients, who need the feedback provided by eye contact and verbal responses from the therapist. Kernberg (1975) recommended a more structured form of psychoanalytic therapy, involving an active technique focusing on confrontations of maladaptive defenses. One wonders whether this technique is useful because it modifies defenses or because it introduces more structure into the therapy. Any form of therapist activity with borderline patients could be experienced by the patient as structuring feedback that prevents disorganization and regression.

The problems that BPD patients have in the hospital setting are similar to those they can experience in intensive psychotherapy. In both settings it is the ambiguity of the environment that can lead to impulsive acting out. In general, empathy in the absence of structure and clear expectations creates precisely this ambiguity. The intense interpersonal climate of psychodynamic psychotherapy has the capacity to mobilize unmeetable needs in the patient, producing increased dysphoria. Therefore, most therapists treating patients with BPD strongly recommend the consistent setting of limits.

Many of the management problems in outpatient therapies for BPD center around the maintenance of structure and boundaries. Borderline patients may not attend regularly or be on time for sessions, and can have trouble leaving when their time is up. Often they demand an increased frequency of meetings, but they rarely feel "held," no matter how often they are seen. They may insist on access by telephone between sessions, or they may call with suicidal threats at night. Such difficulties are the main reason why borderline patients are often times unpopular with many therapists.

It is possible that these boundary problems, which are also found in the interpersonal relations of the patient, could be intensified by dynamic therapy, in which the uncovering of conflict is emphasized. BPD cases require external structuring until they are able to develop a stable therapeutic alliance. Borderline patients have problems being observers of their own therapy, and their alliances are based more on their needs than on a commitment to work on knowing themselves better (Adler 1985). It has even been suggested that the establishment of a working alliance is not the beginning of therapy with this population, but a goal for the end point of treatment (Adler 1979).

Much of the confusion about the use of intensive therapy in BPD may derive from the existence of subgroups of borderline patients who need different approaches (Waldinger 1987). The more impulsive borderline patients need the most structure, and it is this group who are most likely to drop out of treatment (Gunderson et al. 1989). In these cases, if psychotherapy is attempted, it would have to be modified in favor of increased therapist activity, even to the extent of creating a somewhat more authoritarian climate. It is interesting in this regard that BPD patients may form an important percentage of those attracted to cults (Deutsch 1975). However, therapy need not be cultish for there to be a positive working alliance.

The ultimate goal of any psychotherapy is to target maladaptive behaviors and to replace them with a more adaptive repertoire. Kroll (1988) defines the aim of therapy in BPD as "competence." This term has been widely used in the child development literature to describe behavioral skills that are protective against psychopathology (Garmezy and Rutter 1983). Competence means that the patient can obtain posi-

tive reinforcements for adaptive skills. Although it may not be a sufficient condition for a good therapeutic result, it seems like a necessary
one.

The problem with intensive therapies for BPD is that although the
ultimate aim is competence, some of the strategies for arriving at this
goal can produce regression rather than progression. There may be a
subgroup of borderline patients who tolerate regression, but they would
most likely be those who have important areas of competence outside
the treatment. When present, areas of external competence provide
stable reinforcements that allow the interpersonal world to be dealt with
more constructively.

Stone (1987), in his follow-up study, retrospectively rated borderline patients for their suitability for analytically oriented therapy. He
concluded that only a third had been truly amenable to this treatment,
and this was in a group of patients who had been preselected as suitable.
It is possible that only those borderline patients who have already established some area of competence can benefit from dynamic psychotherapy. Although this hypothesis will have to be documented through
empirical research, it is in accordance with findings from the psychotherapy outcome literature that the patients who benefit most from
therapy are those with the highest level of adaptive functioning (Garfield 1986). Because many BPD patients are functioning at low levels of
competence, it seems likely that only a proportion of BPD cases would
be helped by psychodynamic therapy and that the majority of cases are
not suitable.

There have been few empirical studies of psychodynamic therapy in
BPD. Perhaps the most frequently quoted report of the outcome of
long-term intensive therapy is a study done at the Menninger Clinic
(Kernberg et al. 1972), but its findings are of questionable relevance to
BPD because it examined a small sample who were never formally diagnosed. One recent study (Stevenson and Meares 1992) evaluated the
effectiveness of 1 year of outpatient intensive psychotherapy for a group
of borderline patients. The method was based on object-relations theory, and therapy was conducted at a frequency of twice a week. The
results were encouraging on a number of measures, but there was no
control group and thus there is no way of knowing whether the positive

outcome was attributable to the specific methods used. Nevertheless, this study does show that there is a cohort of borderline patients who respond to dynamic psychotherapy.

The question is how far such results can be generalized to the larger BPD population. The research literature also provides evidence that intensive psychotherapy applied to borderline patients is associated with serious attrition. Over half of BPD patients assigned to open-ended psychotherapy drop out early (Gunderson et al. 1989; Skodol et al. 1983), and BPD patients tend to leave treatment against advice with even the most experienced therapists (Waldinger and Gunderson 1984). These findings could reflect either problems in establishing alliances with borderline patients, the inappropriate use of intensive therapy techniques for less competent patients, or the unrealistic expectations of therapists.

What we need are clinical trials of intensive psychotherapy in BPD. In the meantime, psychodynamic therapy should not be prescribed simply because patients are profoundly troubled or because other therapies have failed. We need to know for sure whether this treatment works and whether it works better than other treatments that use up fewer clinical resources.

Option 4: Cognitive-Behavior Therapy

Beck and Freeman (1990) have described the principles under which cognitive-behavior therapy (CBT), a treatment originally developed for depression, could be applied to patients with personality disorders. CBT is an adaptation of behavior therapy that applies strategies used to change behaviors to the cognitions that accompany maladaptive behavioral responses.

A specific method of CBT for borderline patients has been developed by Linehan (1993), who has based her technical procedures on a theoretical model of BPD. She calls her method "dialectical behavior therapy" (DBT). The term "dialectical" is derived from the philosophy of Hegel, in which opposed principles in dialectic relationship undergo creative synthesis. However, a knowledge of philosophy is not required to understand Linehan's methods on a pragmatic level. The interventions consist of identifying pathological cognitions and maladaptive be-havior patterns in BPD and targeting them for change. In particular, DBT is designed to reduce parasuicidal behaviors, the symptoms that most interfere with therapy and that most compromise the patient's quality of life. In addition, there are techniques in DBT in which pa-tients are taught to manage their emotional states, with impulsivity and affective instability being the target behaviors.

The theory behind DBT is fairly similar to the model presented in this book. In DBT, borderline pathology is seen as arising from an inter-action of a biologically determined emotional vulnerability that is am-plified by a nonvalidating family environment. Although emotional vulnerability is thought to be constitutional, patients can benefit from specific interventions that train them to regulate dysphoria. Learning emotional control obviates the need for impulsive action, and patients are encouraged to understand the emotional reactions that led up to their parasuicidal actions and to examine the alternatives to impulsivity. The therapeutic atmosphere validates patients' emotions, and patients are trained to validate their feelings themselves.

Dialectical behavior therapy is one of the most promising develop-ments in the treatment of BPD. The methods involve a combination of individual and group therapy. In contrast to so many other clini-cians, Linehan has exposed her treatment results to empirical evalua-tion. The first study was a randomized clinical trial in which patients were assigned either to DBT or to "treatment as usual" in the commu-nity (Linehan et al. 1991). DBT is a manualized treatment, and, as mentioned above, its specific interventions are designed to reduce parasuicide. The patients received individual therapy, as well as psy-choeducational group therapy, weekly for 1 year. They were required to commit themselves specifically to a reduction in parasuicide and were taught methods of managing emotional distress, such as behavioral skills training in interpersonal relationships, distress tolerance, and emotional regulation. Although the patients were allowed to telephone their ther-apists rather frequently, this did not seem to lead to a regressive vicious circle, possibly because of the highly structured nature of the treatment. The effectiveness of the therapy was shown by a threefold reduction in instances of parasuicide, whereas in the control group the number of parasuicidal incidents actually increased. Moreover, patients in DBT were more likely to stay in therapy and had fewer hospitalizations. There were no differences between DBT and the control condition on measures of depression, hopelessness, or suicidal ideation. The positive effects were maintained at 1-year follow-up (Linehan et al. 1993). Although DBT is designed primarily for outpatients, there is also a comparative treatment trial being run at New York Hospital with inpatients randomly assigned to units using psychodynamic therapy or DBT (Shearin and Linehan 1993).

This clinical trial of DBT demonstrates that measurable results can be obtained when maladaptive behavior is targeted in BPD. The patients in the study were expected to make a strong commitment to their treatment, and still only 16% of them dropped out, much less than the 50% dropout rate described for dynamic psychotherapy. There remains some question as to whether the results obtained on this sample apply to the BPD population as a whole, and the results require replication in other settings. Another caveat is that in spite of the apparent specificity of DBT, its effectiveness could still be partly nonspecific, resulting from a highly structured treatment provided by strongly committed therapists.

Nevertheless, there seem to be elements in DBT that are specifically effective for BPD. One such specific element could be the cognitive management of intense dysphoria. Another is the structured program of skills training, which resembles the psychoeducational treatments that are known to be effective in schizophrenia (Hogarty et al. 1979).

The main unanswered question is whether the method can produce long-term effects that last beyond the period of treatment. In a follow-up of patients 1 year after the end of treatment, Linehan (1993) found that, compared with the control group, DBT patients maintained their greater improvement, although they continued to be symptomatic. It is possible that DBT, like other psychotherapies for BPD, requires an extended period of time to achieve stable improvement. DBT is an important new development in the management of borderline patients and is the only treatment option to have undergone rigorous clinical trials.

Option 5: Supportive Psychotherapy

The term "supportive psychotherapy" is another psychiatric misnomer, since it fails to define what is being supported. The term was originally intended to distinguish analytic therapy, in which defenses are confronted, from forms of treatment in which a weak ego is supported by discussions on a more practical level. But defining supportive therapy by what it is not does not do justice to this approach. The treatment can be characterized operationally as involving 1) a lower frequency of sessions, usually once a week; 2) a focus on the current life situation of the patient; and 3) an emphasis on the therapeutic alliance rather than on transference.

Zetzel (1971), a psychoanalyst impressed by the fragility of borderline patients and their tendency to regress in treatment, advocated a once-weekly contact that is more containing than exploratory. Zetzel and also Friedman (1975) have recommended supportive therapy for BPD based on a critique of the problems that can emerge in intensive psychotherapy.

A useful model for supportive therapy is to define the primary task of treatment as the development of competence (Kroll 1988). A reasonably detailed model of this therapy, based on psychodynamic principles, has been described by Rockland (1992). Some of the techniques parallel those of DBT. By meeting regularly with a therapist who validates emotions, the patient learns to modulate dysphoria and to regulate the tendency to respond to problems with impulsive action. Much of the discussion focuses on problems in relationships with others, and patients are taught to manage interpersonal relations with a greater tolerance for difficulties. Supportive therapy, therefore, has a psychoeducational component.

In practice, supportive psychotherapy may be the most frequently used form of treatment for BPD. Borderline patients who come to outpatient clinics, community mental health centers, or private offices are often offered supportive therapy in some form because this modality does not use up large resources. It is also possible to combine elements of intensive dynamic therapy with supportive therapy, depending on the ego strength of the patient (Rockland 1992).

Supportive therapy need not necessarily continue indefinitely, but there seem to be some patients who end up becoming quite dependent on it. Horwitz (1974) described such a group of personality disorder patients from the Menninger study who were jocularly known as "lifers." Knowledge of the long-term outcome of BPD suggests a useful alternative. Borderline patients may benefit as much from intermittent as from continuous therapy (S. Perry 1989). When we consider the chronicity of the disorder, it makes sense to establish a strong working alliance, institute active treatment, and then wean the patient off regular therapy, while keeping the door open for management of future crises. When patients are discharged, they retain easy and readily available access to the therapist whenever they are in difficulty. This approach may not suit therapists who like a regular schedule with filled hours, but it could be of particular value to patients in controlling regression and maximizing autonomy. It is probably not coincidental that some of the researchers involved in studying the long-term outcome of BPD were initially advocates of intensive psychotherapy but were convinced by their own research results that long-term intermittent treatment should be considered the standard method for BPD (McGlashan 1993; Silver 1983, 1985).

The intermittent therapy model acknowledges that BPD, like the major functional psychoses or like many medical conditions, is a chronic illness. A reasonable expectation for patients with such disorders is to encourage them to leave active treatment when they improve but to leave the door open. Therapeutic holidays were originally recommended by Alexander and French (1946) as a means of combatting regression in long-term psychotherapy. This method could have a special value for borderline patients.

Another variant of intermittent therapy is crisis intervention. There seem to be borderline patients who never develop a therapeutic alliance but who still need an entry point into the mental health care system. Clinicians will be familiar with those individuals who generally appear only in emergency rooms, and then perhaps for a few crisis visits thereafter. Perhaps these individuals constitute a subgroup of BPD patients who cannot tolerate a therapeutic relationship.

Option 6: Group Therapy

Group therapy in BPD could be considered as another form of supportive treatment and has many of the same goals. The primary difference is that the group performs the functions assigned to the therapist in individual therapy, and its effects on patients may be the result of different mechanisms than those in individual therapy. As described by Munroe-Blum (1992), the purposes of group therapy in BPD are to provide modeling of social roles, to apply peer pressure, and to offer a holding environment. The group setting dilutes transference and tends to avoid some of its difficulties. It could be used for homogeneous BPD groups, as in DBT, or for mixed groups of patients. Group therapy has been used in outpatient clinics, but has been most frequently applied in inpatient or day centers, for the practical reason that patients are already involved in a common experience.

The theory of group therapy (Yalom 1985) is that it confronts patients with maladaptive behaviors in a context where better responses can be learned. The problem in applying this method to BPD is that the group by itself may be insufficiently supportive in the short run to contain the dysphoria seen in the BPD patient, so that the drop-out rate with group treatment alone could be high. For this reason, group therapy is often used as an adjunct to individual treatment, as has been suggested by Linehan (1993).

There is one controlled clinical trial in progress of group therapy as a primary modality (Munroe-Blum 1992). This trial is using a treatment called relationship management therapy (RMT; Dawson and MacMillan 1993), a method whose technique emphasizes the importance of therapists avoiding becoming entangled in the pathological expectations of the borderline patient.

Option 7: No Treatment

There seem to be BPD patients who are better off without any treatment (Frances et al. 1984; Friedman 1975). This subgroup is self-selected in that they respond so negatively to therapy that they either avoid it entirely or drop out early. For such patients, who usually have paranoid trends in their personality, the complications of therapy could create too much distress to make the process worth their while. Clinicians should keep this possibility in mind, particularly because so many BPD patients do not show dramatic benefits from existing forms of treatment.

Mechanisms for the Successful Treatment of Borderline Personality Disorder

One way of understanding how treatment aids recovery in BPD is to consider its effect on the dimensions of the disorder. The basic theory of this book is that personality traits such as impulsivity and affective lability underlie BPD and that negative environmental factors amplify these traits to pathological proportions. Therefore, there are two possible ways to intervene to reverse this process: 1) directly modify traits and/or 2) change the amplifying environment.

Symptomatic interventions target those clinical phenomena that reflect the traits underlying BPD. Whether these interventions involve psychopharmacology, full or partial hospitalization, or psychotherapy, damping down impulsivity and affective instability is the primary task of treatment. But these effects could be temporary if they do not influence the patient's environment. This environment, which consists primarily of the current interpersonal relations of the patient, has to be changed. The process could be conceptualized as reversing the amplification of traits to a disorder. It involves breaking vicious circles that develop between the core dimensions, because impulsive actions often lead to the breakup of relationships, which in turn makes the patient more dysphoric and then more impulsive.

Changing the patient's interpersonal environment may be one mechanism that explains why psychotherapy could be useful in the treatment of BPD. If a stressful environment were responsible for amplifying traits, then a soothing one could damp them down. The process usually starts in the therapeutic relationship, but treatment also has to actively encourage environmental changes to make relationships validating for the patient. As has been pointed out by several authors on the process of psychotherapy (Alexander and French 1946; Wachtel 1977), most of the process of working through emotional conflicts takes place in significant relationships outside of treatment.

For many borderline patients, their interpersonal environment replicates the worst aspects of their early psychological experiences. Patients with BPD make poor object choices, and many of the important people in their life are in fact hurtful or neglectful. But not all borderline patients will be able to change their relationships so as to make adequate and satisfying choices. What most patients can learn is at least to avoid the most pathological interpersonal situations and to obtain reinforcements in other sectors of their life, such as work.

Borderline patients who have been successfully treated retain some of their underlying traits. They are inclined to react emotionally to life situations and to act impulsively on their feelings. However, when these traits are not amplified to a high intensity, they are not automatic responses to any stressful situation. At this level, personality traits need no longer interfere with interpersonal functioning.

These hypothesized mechanisms for successful treatment of BPD are consistent with the biopsychosocial model proposed in this book. First, the biological dimensions behind BPD are the ultimate targets of symptomatic treatment. Second, understanding the psychological risk factors for BPD can lead us to interventions designed to help borderline patients stop recreating pathogenic situations in their present life. Finally, when the role of the social environment in BPD is taken into consideration, it follows that treatments need sufficient structure to be workable.

Having described the possible mechanisms of successful treatment, we must acknowledge that the treatment of BPD is far from being necessarily successful. Based on existing research findings (Kernberg et al. 1972), the patients who respond best to treatment will be those with greater premorbid competence. As Horwitz (1974) archly commented, "The rich get richer and the poor get poorer."

Finally, we need not be upset that characteristics in the borderline patient are more important for success than is the skill of the therapist. The scarce resources available should be allotted to more treatable cases. As pointed out by one experienced therapist of borderline patients (Kernberg 1975), if one is considering spending years with a patient, one owes it to oneself to choose a patient who can benefit from the investment. There is no reason for therapists to blame themselves for lack of success with borderline patients, or to assume that if only a more experienced or charismatic colleague had been in charge, things would have gone well.

A further implication of baseline differences among borderline patients in premorbid functioning is that there may be different optimal management strategies for different BPD subgroups. In view of the finding of outcome research that there is wide variation in long-term course, ranging from intractability to dramatic recovery, there are important clinical implications to the heterogeneity of BPD populations. We need to identify subgroups phenomenologically and then to match them with different treatment modalities (Waldinger 1987).

Summary

We are just beginning to have empirical data on which to base treatment planning for borderline patients. At present, any conclusions must be highly tentative. However, based on the evidence summarized in this chapter, the following points can be made:

1. There is no definitive treatment for BPD.
2. There are no clear-cut predictors of which borderline patients will best respond to treatment.
3. When borderline patients do respond to treatment, the results are not necessarily specific to the therapeutic intervention used.
4. The most useful treatments target the dimension of impulsivity in BPD.
5. Borderline patients can benefit from learning how to regulate their emotional lability.
6. Borderline patients do better in treatments that provide clear boundaries, limits, and structures.
7. Although full or partial hospitalization has a role in treatment, most borderline patients are best managed in outpatient therapy.

8. Outpatient therapy with the borderline patient will in most cases be supportive and oriented toward the patient's interpersonal environment.
9. Treatment of borderline patients can be intermittent.
10. Most cases of BPD will require some form of follow-up after termination of regular therapy.

In the next chapter we apply some of these principles to a general plan for the clinical management of borderline patients.

9

Clinical Management

In Chapter 8 we provided a cross-sectional survey of the treatment options for borderline personality disorder. In the present chapter we examine the clinical management of BPD in a longitudinal perspective. We will define the principles of treatability, discuss how to select among treatment options for different patients, describe the course and goals of therapy, and present an approach to posttermination follow-up.

Guidelines for Clinical Management

The overall guidelines for clinical management will be based on the literature reviewed in the previous chapter. In principle, any rational approach to therapy should be well grounded in clinical trials and should provide a link between research and practice. However, there is an enormous gulf between our empirical knowledge and the practical problems of treating borderline patients. There has been very little research on the value of specific interventions in the course of treatment. Clinical trials are more useful in helping choose modalities of therapy than in guiding the conduct of treatment in detail.

Therefore, in this chapter the strongly empirical point of view of this book will have to be relaxed, and many assertions will be presented that cannot yet be backed up by research findings. Instead, multiple clinical vignettes will be used to demonstrate the principles of treat-

133

ment. Although the guidelines presented in this chapter are based ultimately on clinical experience, they are reasonably consistent with the findings presented in Chapter 8 and can be considered as hypotheses suitable for future empirical testing.

The approach to clinical management in this chapter will be an integrative eclecticism that takes into account biological, psychological, and social factors. Treatment recommendations will be consistent with a multidimensional point of view. Because outpatient therapy is the mainstay of management for BPD, the majority of the vignettes and discussion focus on treatment in clinic settings.

The following guidelines are used to describe the stages of evaluation, treatment, and follow-up of borderline patients:

1. Each patient must be first assessed for treatability.
2. The first aim of treatment is the control of symptoms.
3. Borderline patients require structure.
4. The ultimate aim of treatment is competence.
5. Treatment in BPD is usually intermittent.

Determining Treatability

Borderline patients vary widely in their treatability, and every patient needs to be carefully evaluated before initiating therapy. The pretreatment assessment is a triage in which patients will fall into three groups: those who are untreatable, those who require primarily support and crisis intervention, and those who can benefit from more extensive psychotherapy. Triage is important in applying scarce resources rationally and effectively.

Fortunately, few borderline patients are untreatable. As discussed in Chapter 8, there are patients who are too suspicious to form a treatment alliance. Such cases tend to be seen in emergency settings. Most of them will be lost to follow-up after the emergency assessment. But sometimes these patients can be offered treament that leads to complications. The first vignette demonstrates such a case.

Vignette 1

A 23-year-old woman presented repeatedly to the emergency room of a general hospital. She was unable to have any close relationships, and she would visit the hospital when she felt empty and lonely, complaining of suicidal feelings. Her interviews with the psychiatrist on call developed a malignant pattern. Although she would begin by talking about her depression, in a short time she would become angry and suspicious about almost any line of questioning. These feelings would then escalate until the patient became physically assaultive. The first few times this happened, she was held in the hospital under civil commitment. However, on each of these occasions her suicidal mood quickly abated and she asked to be released the next day. As her behavior became well known to the emergency staff, it became a matter of policy not to admit her.

This patient was seen 12 years later as part of a follow-up study of BPD patients. She was unemployed and socially isolated. Her attempts to get involved in therapy had been unsuccessful because of her suspiciousness.

This vignette describes a patient for whom treatment resources may have been misapplied. But untreatability is a state, not a trait. Impulsivity in BPD usually declines over time, and when patients are no longer as impulsive, they may become more accessible. This patient was an exception to this rule, because she had paranoid traits that continued to interfere with treatability even when her impulsive actions declined.

The majority of borderline patients accept, at least initially, a reasonable treatment plan. But, as discussed in the previous chapter, many of them drop out of therapy after a few months. The question is whether dropouts reflect treatment failures or bad prescriptions.

The therapeutic alliances of borderline patients are fragile (Frank 1992). Two studies (Gunderson et al. 1989; Skodol et al. 1983) have shown that over half of borderline patients will be early dropouts from psychotherapy. The clinical challenge is to predict the severity of problems in alliance formation. Unfortunately, this is a notably difficult thing to do. In a study of psychotherapy with a wide variety of patients, Luborsky (1988) found that the strength of the alliance strongly predicts therapy outcome, but that it can only be reliably measured after patients have already had a few sessions of treatment. He therefore recommends trying a course of psychotherapy on any patient willing to undertake it, and simply waiting to see how things turn out. This might be a reasonable approach for many patients, but it seems an impractical way to determine treatability in BPD. With borderline patients, after only a few sessions of therapy, one may be faced with escalating impulsivity and unmanageable transference. At that point there are enough data to come to a decision, but it is difficult to disengage from the patient.

Ego strength could predict alliance formation and, therefore, treatability. This construct can be operationally defined as the level of functioning in work and relationships prior to treatment. As reviewed in Chapter 8, ego strength was the best predictor of outcome in the Menninger study (Kernberg et al. 1972). In that study, the main mechanism of successful treatment was alliance formation (Horwitz 1974).

The most predictive aspect of pretreatment functioning for therapy could be the capacity to work. Treatment is also work and requires a great deal of persistence. Patients do not improve unless they come regularly and apply themselves to the task at hand. Patients who have not remained on any job for more than a few months are likely to act similarly in treatments that require frustration tolerance. Because work is a structured task with fairly clear boundaries, there are many borderline patients who show surprising competence on the job. This ability to maintain commitment to tasks in the workplace or at school can be used to evaluate treatability. Measuring ego strength in homemakers can be somewhat more complex. Family life has less intrinsic structure, and homemakers have to create one. Some borderline patients who stay home with children have serious difficulties carrying out the tasks of parenting in a predictable way (M. Weiss, P. Zelkowitz, J. Vogel, et al, manuscript submitted for publication).

Another possible predictor of alliance formation is how patients have behaved with other significant persons in their life. Because the ability to benefit from psychotherapy depends on tolerating closeness and feeling trust, the capacity for intimacy could be evaluated from analogous situations in the patient's past life. Borderline patients have serious problems in interpersonal relationships, but those who have been involved for some time in an intimate relationship, even a troubled one, might be more easily helped than those who have not. If, for example, a patient has been unable to manage any meaningful relationship (as was the case for the patient in Vignette 1), he or she is less likely to manage one with a psychotherapist. The presence of loyal friendships could also be a positive prognostic sign. For some patients, although difficulties arise in intimate or romantic attachments, bonding can be tolerated in settings that have structure and where limits have been set. Therapy is such a setting.

Given the nature of borderline pathology, intimate relationships are the setting in which the most pathological behavior occurs. One sees patients with BPD who can work but cannot manage intimacy, but not patients who have achieved intimacy but cannot work. This is another reason why work is a more practical predictor of treatment response.

Baseline ego strength could also be used as a clinical guideline to treatment assignment. By definition, borderline patients are deficient in ego strength. But there is a good deal of variability among patients meeting BPD criteria on the quality of their work and their relationships. Borderline patients who can benefit from intensive psychotherapy could be those who can hold a job or follow an educational program, and those who have at least attempted to establish intimate relationships. Other patients could be assigned to more supportive therapy if they have been chronically unemployed and/or unable to establish relationships. Many borderline patients are most comfortable with intermittent supportive contact and crisis interventions, and we can capitalize on this phenomenon rather than routinely offer forms of therapy that most patients cannot tolerate.

Let us consider as examples two patients, both of whom had serious borderline psychopathology but who fell on opposite ends of the spectrum of ego strength.

Vignette 2

A 23-year-old student presented with suicidal ideas following a failed long-term love affair. She functioned well at the university and was preparing for a professional career. Although she had made several unwise choices in her intimate relations, she had strong friends of both sexes with whom she maintained long-term and meaningful contact.

She remained in intensive psychotherapy for 5 years. Her heterosexual relationships continued to be marked by emotional turmoil, and the course of treatment was equally stormy. She made one serious suicide attempt and was continuously suicidal for almost the entire course of the therapy. She often left her therapist unsure if she would survive from one appointment to the next.

However, the ultimate outcome was quite satisfactory. She was able to make use of her pretreatment ego strengths to become successful in her professional life. Possibly as a result of learning to trust the therapist, she made a good marriage, after which she was no longer suicidal. At 5-year follow-up, her career had remained on track, and she was a competent mother of two children.

Vignette 3

One 32-year-old man had never held a steady job and survived on social welfare. In his younger years he had cruised in gay bars without forming enduring relationships. As he grew older, he attempted to establish intimate relationships, but when, after a few months, each affair ended, he would slash his wrists.

This patient had attended several outpatient clinics around the city. When he was followed regularly in supportive therapy, his impulsivity was curbed, but each time that he found a new lover he would interrupt treatment. He had been treated with several types of antidepressants without notable success. He was managed in a crisis clinic, where he would usually be seen for a few sessions to contain his dysphoria after parasuicidal episodes.

In these examples both patients had severe borderline psychopathology and both presented a significant risk of suicide. However, they differed in their capacity to develop a working alliance and to make use of a therapeutic relationship. Ego strength may reflect the capacity to benefit from the most active ingredient of psychotherapy, the "nonspecific factors" associated with the therapeutic alliance. The patient in Vignette 2 had high ego strength and was able to work both at her profession and at the tasks of therapy. She was therefore able to benefit from a relationship with a therapist in spite of the extent of her psychopathology. The patient described in Vignette 3 had low ego strength and was not able to work consistently at a job or in treatment. He therefore could not tolerate therapeutic relationships for long and was best managed with multiple crisis interventions.

Symptom Control

Borderline patients come to treatment with prominent and disturbing symptoms. Those symptoms that lie on the impulsive dimension can be disruptive to the treatment structure itself. Unless impulsivity is brought under control, it may be impossible to address other issues. This does not mean that patients are expected simply to give up their symptoms. Linehan's (1993) approach strikes the right note: patients must commit themselves to curbing their parasuicidal actions, but they are not expected to stop until an alliance is established.

A distinction can be made between impulsive symptoms that interfere with treatment and those that do not. Impulsivity outside therapy can be tolerated, but impulsivity inside therapy disrupts the alliance and prevents useful work from being done. For example, if a patient comes regularly to sessions, talks about the circumstances of a failed relationship, but describes having made several small cuts with a razor blade on the wrist after a quarrel and then states that suicide is the only solution, we have a normative situation for the therapy of BPD. If, on the other hand, a patient either comes to sessions intoxicated or fails entirely to come to sessions, and then calls up the therapist repeatedly in the middle of the night threatening suicide, then it is hard to see how therapy can proceed.

The most common impulsive symptom in BPD is parasuicide. Overdoses and wrist slashing can arouse a good deal of concern among therapists. To be worried is not unwarranted, because 1 in 10 borderline patients eventually commit suicide. But, as discussed in the last two chapters, there is no evidence that there are any specific interventions that prevent suicide in BPD. What could be reassuring for therapists of borderline patients is the finding reported in Chapter 7 that the largest number of completed suicides take place after failed treatments, rather than occurring in the midst of therapy. The risk is therefore probably lower if the patient is engaged in treatment, no matter how intense her or his dysphoria. With this principle in mind, suicidality need not be considered an obstacle to the development of a working alliance. In fact, too much concern about a fatal outcome may deflect treatment from its ultimate goals. Suicidality "goes with the territory" of BPD, and even the most suicidal patients can be treated as outpatients.

Interventions to control impulsivity depend on the specific nature of the symptomatology. The control of substance abuse may require specific rehabilitation programs. As discussed in Chapter 8, when life-threatening suicide attempts take place, brief hospitalization is generally indicated. For parasuicidal events such as mild overdoses and self-mutilation, the hospital setting is of doubtful value, and most of these episodes can be handled in clinic settings. When impulsivity is out of control, an alternative to admission is the use of partial hospitalization. Day programs offer sufficient protection and allow close enough observation to institute new forms of treatment when outpatient management has failed.

There are several interventions, described in the previous chapter, that have been shown to control impulsivity in BPD. They do not necessarily require hospitalization for their implementation. Low-dose neuroleptics are often worth a trial; their effects are measurably helpful if not dramatic. There are also psychotherapeutic programs that target impulsive symptomatology, such as dialectical behavior therapy (DBT) or psychoeducation (Silk et al. 1992). The day hospital is a good place to introduce these modalities, and the setting also has a useful nonspecific effect. Most programs involve structured activity of various kinds over the course of the day, so that there are no unstructured times during which patients can regress, as they can when fully admitted.

Many borderline patients are seriously noncompliant with treatment. They will not attend day hospital even if their impulsivity escalates. There are two possibilities when the chaos around borderline patients is not under control. The first would be full hospitalization. If, in spite of its risks, admission is chosen, there should at least be some specific plan for symptom control, whether psychopharmacological or psychoeducational. The alternative would be to decide that at this particular point the patient is not treatable. One would not want to make such a decision after a life-threatening overdose. But it might be quite reasonable to discontinue active treatment with noncompliant patients with uncontrolled substance abuse and parasuicidal gestures.

The following examples demonstrate contrasting situations in which brief admission was applied effectively and ineffectively.

Vignette 4

A 16-year-old high school student presented for treatment after the death by suicide of her best friend. The other girl, who had also been treated for BPD at the same clinic, had in fact suggested a suicide pact with the patient, and then jumped off a bridge.

The presenting patient was suicidal in her own right and had recurrent episodes of wrist slashing. She also had significant micropsychotic symptoms, in particular the intense fantasy that her life was a dream and that she was living on another planet, where she had another existence and a real family. She thought that if she were to die, she would wake up and return to her true home. She would hear the voices of individual characters in this fantasy speaking to her and asking her to join them.

Her social supports were less than ideal. She was living with her older sister, since having run away both from her alcoholic mother and from her father, who had incestuously abused her. Both her parents remained disturbingly present in her life.

The patient was seen for a year in weekly outpatient psychotherapy, which she attended regularly. However, on the anniversary of her friend's death, the patient developed a strong fantasy that she must join her, and indicated to her therapist that she could not control this impulse. Her subsequent hospitalization lasted a month and achieved several purposes. It carried the patient over the ominous anniversary. Family therapy was carried out to support her sister and brother-in-law and to help the patient keep her distance from her parents. The patient was put on trifluoperazine, which controlled her cognitive symptoms. She was then followed in outpatient therapy for another year. [The outcome of this case will be discussed later in this chapter.]

Vignette 5

A 23-year-old unemployed woman was briefly admitted on several occasions for suicidal threats. On each occasion she developed increasing symptoms within 24 hours after hospitalization. After talking about her diffculties to one of the nursing staff, she would slash her wrists. Self-mutilation occurred very rarely outside the hospital and would stop when she was discharged. The patient was eventually managed with multiple crisis interventions until her impulsivity lessened with time.

The first example demonstrates how hospitalization can be used to support outpatient treatment. There were specific treatment plans for the admission, and the hospital setting achieved symptom control through the use of a variety of modalities. In the second example, there was no plan for the management of chronic suicidality other than holding and observation. The patient in Vignette 5 had much lower ego strength and tended to regress in an unstructured ward environment rather than make use of its resources.

In the following example, the structured environment of a day program was helpful in bringing impulsive symptoms under control.

Vignette 6

A 44-year-old unemployed man had been in psychiatric treatment for 27 years, during which he had been treated intermittently, either with crisis intervention, antidepressants, or supportive follow-up. He was referred to the day hospital when he slashed his wrists in the office of his therapist.

The treatment consisted mainly of occupational therapy and a low dose of chlorpromazine. The patient attended faithfully and participated in all scheduled activities, and 8 weeks later, his symptoms dramatically abated. He was then followed as an outpatient, requiring readmission to the day center with similar symptoms 18 months later.

The stabilizing effects of day hospitalization for parasuicide in this patient were largely due to a highly structured environment. The effects were temporary but valuable for management of a very chronic and poorly functioning patient.

Even in the outpatient therapy setting, there can be enough structure and support to achieve symptom control. There is usually a lag period before the effect "kicks in," because it takes time for borderline patients to develop a therapeutic alliance. Although the alliance is fragile at the beginning of treatment, it usually becomes stronger with time. As patients begin to feel comfortable with a therapist and work on their problems, dysphoria abates and there is less need for impulsive action.

The next two vignettes demonstrate how the therapeutic alliance in outpatient psychotherapy controls symptoms.

Vignette 7

A 24-year-old graduate student presented with difficulties in finishing her thesis. She had been previously treated in her home city for her symptoms, including frequent wrist slashing, vivid auditory hallucinations, and mood swings.

The patient began to attend psychotherapy twice a week. She was initially quite suspicious of the therapist, and it took about 6 months to establish a good alliance. At that point both the parasuicidal impulses and the micropsychosis disappeared entirely. When she returned to her home city to pursue her studies, she again began to hear voices and slash her wrists. These symptoms continued until she obtained a new therapist, when they again subsided.

In this case, the symptoms, although at times alarming, were never life threatening. This patient had in fact good social supports. It was important not to interfere with the patient's area of highest competence, her graduate studies, and therefore to provide outpatient treatment. Her symptoms came readily under control as soon as she formed a working alliance.

Vignette 8

A 19-year-old student in her second semester at the university presented with wrist slashing, mood swings, uncontrollable rages, and continuous depersonalization. She was initially quite reticent with her male therapist. In these first few months her depersonalization and wrist slashing increased. She made a long-distance call to an affective disorders clinic in another city and was told that she was getting the wrong treatment and that she should be on an antidepressant. This episode did not really endanger the therapy, and within a few months she began to develop a working alliance.

Whereas in the past she had always insisted that there was nothing wrong with her family, she now began to provide a meaningful history of her childhood. It emerged that her father had been hospitalized for a psychosis, and although he had recovered, he remained a violent and frightening man. Although there had been no sexual or physical abuse, her memories of life in the family were full of terror. Her mother, who was chronically ill, had been unable to protect her. The patient, an only child, had retreated into a world of fantasy in her room.

As she told her story, she became attached to the therapist, whom she began to see as kind and paternal. At the same time her symptoms vanished. The rest of the therapy concerned her need to separate herself from her elderly but still difficult parents and her need to open herself to intimate relationships in the present. On 2-year follow-up she was living on the opposite coast, working regularly, and involved for the first time in a serious heterosexual relationship.

Lasting control of impulsive symptoms in BPD takes time. As discussed in Chapter 7, these symptoms decrease as patients age, but treatment may have an effect in shortening the recovery time. There are many borderline patients with complex histories of treatment from different therapists. It is possible, as suggested by Wolberg (1973), that splitting defenses in borderline patients make multiple therapies an inevitable part of the process of recovery. More likely, patients become more treatable as the disorder abates naturalistically. In the following example, recovery occurred only after therapy was broken off and resumed.

Vignette 9

A 22-year-old woman presented for therapy because of intense suicidal ideation and disturbed interpersonal relationships. Although she was notably competent in her profession and had good friends, her intimate attachments with men were highly problematical. Several of her boyfriends were criminals, and she had hidden them from the police at her apartment. Her childhood was marked by the death of her mother when she was 7. Her alcoholic father had been unable to look after her, and she had entered foster care. Although the foster parents were religious and highly devoted people, she found them cold and had the fantasy that her father would return to rescue her.

She attended regular psychotherapy for 3 years. In the course of this time, she never ceased to be intensely suicidal. She felt out of control of her life and needed to know that if necessary she could end it. In order to spare the therapist the burden of her symptoms, she would call suicide hotlines in the middle of the night to talk anonymously.

A crisis arose when she at length decided to seek out her father and found him to be a chronic alcoholic with little interest in her. A few weeks later she became depressed with a number of delusional ideas. She was briefly hospitalized and treated with low-dose neuroleptics, which controlled her psychotic thinking. However, she felt disillusioned with her therapist, who had not protected her from these complications, and was followed intermittently for the next year by the psychiatrist who treated her in the hospital.

A year later, after the death of her father, she returned to her first therapist, whom she now acknowledged had been another loved and disappointing parent for her. As she discussed this issue, her suicidality disappeared. Six months later she terminated therapy but kept in touch for the next 10 years with Christmas cards. On 15-year follow-up she was working in another city and was involved in a long-term intimate relationship.

This vignette demonstrates several points of clinical interest. The first is that in some patients chronic suicidality not only is part of their borderline psychopathology but performs an important psychological function. The second is that tolerating such suicidality is part of the equipment of the psychotherapist who is comfortable working with borderline patients. This patient, like the one described in Vignette 2, did well in spite of being at serious risk. Nor did psychotic complications predict a poor outcome; as with the patients in vignettes 4 and 7, such symptoms resolved in the course of treatment. The case in Vignette 9 shows that when there is a reasonable working alliance, and when psychological work can be done, symptoms will come under control.

In summary, there seem to be many routes to the control of symptomatology in BPD. Some patients require partial or full hospitalization for short periods of time. In these settings symptom control could be aided by psychopharmacological support or psychoeducational programs. In most patients symptoms can be managed on an outpatient basis. Developing a working alliance, teaching patients how to control their emotions, providing support through a trusting relationship, and working through conflicts all function together to achieve the same goal.

The Role of Structure in Treatment

There is an intrinsic structure to well-managed psychotherapy. First, the treatment environment itself is predictable, with a schedule and clear rules of procedure. Second, the tasks to be achieved in therapy are defined rather than undefined.

As we saw in Chapter 4, many borderline patients grow up in families that are chaotic and unstructured. As discussed in Chapter 5, an unstructured social environment may also be a risk factor for BPD. It follows that therapeutic interventions for borderline patients need to maximize structure. Doing so helps contain impulsivity and reduce dysphoria. The ego weakness of the borderline patient reflects an unstructured inner world that requires external strengthening.

In Chapter 8 this principle was applied to understanding some of the complications that can arise in the therapy of BPD patients. Unstructured settings, in which the only expectation is that feelings should be verbalized, can be dangerous for patients who can express emotions but have difficulty in containing them. The success of cognitive-behavioral methods could be in part attributable to their high degree of structure. Similarly, many psychodynamic therapists experienced with BPD (Kernberg 1975) have emphasized limit setting and structuring as preliminary conditions for work on conflict resolution.

The following vignette demonstrates how the level of structure affects treatment. It also reflects the complications associated with the multiple therapies we have seen in the other vignettes in this chapter.

Vignette 10

A 26-year-old woman had been in therapy since mid-adolescence. Her main symptoms were intense hypochondriasis bordering on delusions, and parasuicidal acts. Although in the past she had been treated by three experienced psychiatrists, she had done poorly with all of them. Her treatment during her university years was particularly disastrous, marked by multiple admissions to the hospital and abandonment by her therapist.

Her fourth psychiatrist had begun with a strong commitment, saw her at least 2 to 3 times per week, and permitted her to call him at home whenever she was upset. Over the next 2 years he became "burnt out" with her demands. Moreover, she did not improve as a result of his availability and devotion. After a hospital admission for an overdose, he concluded that she was untreatable and told her she would not benefit from further therapy.

She was then treated by a fifth psychiatrist. He deliberately chose to see her once a week, but she frequently called him in a panic between sessions. He set down the rule that she was allowed one phone call per week. The very next week she phoned twice. The second call opened with the remark, "I'm calling to tell you that I'm about to kill myself." The therapist, who by this point felt confident in his evaluation of this patient's suicidality, replied, "You know you have to wait until the next session to talk about it," and ended the conversation. After this incident the suicidal threats tapered off, but she continued to have micropsychotic symptoms that only partially responded to neuroleptic treatment.

The patient moved to another city and started therapy with a sixth psychiatrist, which lasted for another 3 years. Although she was seen twice a week, no other contact was permitted. The treatment focused on her current interpersonal problems, and she was taken off all her medication. On 10-year follow-up the patient was successful in a professional career and was married with two children. She had residual hypochondriasis, but without the panic that had previously accompanied these symptoms.

It is not entirely clear in this case whether the last therapist was the most skilled or whether the patient had partially recovered with time and become more treatable. Nevertheless, it seems likely that unstructured responses from at least one of her earlier therapists had led to regression.

What makes it difficult to maintain structure in the treatment of BPD is the therapist's perfectly rational concern about the patient's suicidality. How does one keep the rules when the patient states that only by breaking them can her or his life be saved? It seems worth emphasizing again that the equipment of the therapist of a borderline patient includes a certain sangfroid. We simply do not know whether we can prevent these patients from completing suicide; for every case in which one feels that a response was life saving, there are any number of counterexamples in which inaction left the patient resentfully alive. Because treatment easily becomes chaotic when structure is lost, one might conceptualize therapy of BPD as analogous to a risky medical treatment for a potentially fatal disease. One must accept risk to treat patients effectively.

Competence as the Aim of Treatment

Competence refers to the capacity to master life tasks. It was originally introduced as a concept by researchers in child development in the study of children who functioned well in spite of adverse circumstances ("resilient children") (Garmezy and Rutter 1983). The elements that compose competence are the same as those that define ego strength: work and intimate relationships. A competence-oriented approach to treatment has the corollary that more emphasis is put on present functioning than on past traumas. In a psychodynamic model the working through of past experiences is seen as the precondition for better functioning in the present. This approach is implicit in all descriptions of psychoanalytical psychotherapy for borderline patients (Adler 1985;

Kernberg 1984). Moreover, recent evidence for childhood trauma in BPD has led to suggestions that treatment emphasize the integration of such experiences (J. C. Perry 1991). The view presented here is that these models have not been shown to be effective in a wide range of borderline patients and can be associated with a risk of regression. The model being offered in this chapter resembles much more the competence-oriented approach suggested by Kroll (1988) or the cognitive-behavioral approach of Linehan (1993). In terms of the options reviewed in Chapter 8, it could be described as a theoretically informed type of eclectic and supportive psychotherapy.

Just as competence can be used to predict treatability, it could also be a marker to evaluate the results of treatment. Clinicians need to establish goals for therapy and to assess when these goals have been adequately met and treatment can be terminated. The termination point will be different for each patient depending on her or his capacities. Initial ego strength can be used to determine how far a patient can reasonably progress and when a law of diminishing returns is setting in. One sometimes hears that borderline patients are interminable, but excessively long treatments for borderline patients could be an artifact of unrealistic therapeutic goals. Competence is a better measure than cure.

Work may be the most clinically relevant sector of competence. In outcome research, it has been found that most BPD patients do better if they can work (McGlashan 1993). For some patients, work allows them to protect themselves from their pathology by providing a source of satisfaction outside of intimate relationships. In many such cases, patients learn, in fact, to limit their intimate involvements (Bardenstein and McGlashan 1989).

Outcome research in BPD shows that as impulsivity declines, patients become relatively asymptomatic with time (see Chapter 7). But a troubled dynamic core can still be found in recovered borderline patients (Silver and Cardish 1991). Their psychopathology can potentially be reactivated, particularly in an intimate relationship. For many patients there are two solutions to this dilemma: 1) establish a relationship with another person who is tolerant of dependency but who contains the patient's tendency to regress, or 2) avoid intimate relationships. The most successful cases, such as the patients in Vignettes 2 and 4, are able to manage a stable relationship. Many patients, as indicated by the follow-up studies, choose the second option and become more isolated. In the Chestnut Lodge study, men were more easily able to redirect their energies into a work situation, whereas the women continued to have difficulties with intimacy even when they had largely recovered from BPD (Bardenstein and McGlashan 1989).

The following examples demonstrate the importance of the development of competence in BPD, particularly in those patients with a restricted capacity for intimacy.

Vignette 11

A 22-year-old graduate student presented with wrist slashing, repetitive overdoses, and tempestuous relationships with men. Her childhood had been marked by neglect, with a large family left directionless after the early death of her father. There had also been an isolated but dynamically important incident of sexual abuse at age 5, which she had been unable to disclose to her harried mother.

This patient had a suspicious and sarcastic manner, and tolerated therapy with difficulty. She discharged herself at the end of each crisis period, taking the sessions like bad-tasting medicine that would go down if swallowed quickly. Intimacy disorganized her, and after one disappointing relationship, she took a large overdose of pills. For many months thereafter she heard voices asking her to die, which were silenced only by taking trifluoperazine. Over time she decided that she could not handle closeness and that she needed to live alone. She was successful in her studies and became a teacher.

Vignette 12

The patient was first seen in therapy when he dropped out of school at age 18. He had been a good student in high school, but seemed unable to handle the demands of his first year at the university. Behind his inability to manage this developmental transition was a family history in which his brother was physically disabled, his father died young, and his preoccupied mother was left to manage the family. From the age of 18 to 20 the patient had major difficulties with substance abuse and had dominating but unstable relationships with women. He searched for an elusive masculinity by keeping piranha fish and two ferocious dogs. When he felt he could not achieve any of his goals in life, he seriously considered suicide and began wrist slashing. In this phase of his life, therapy was not successful. He became housebound and withdrawn, eventually dropping out of treatment entirely.

Three years later the patient went back to the same therapist and also reentered the university as a mature student. He became involved with a woman classmate who had similar problems, moved in with her within a few weeks, and stopped treatment. This relationship lasted 2 years and ended in a traumatic separation that brought the patient back for a third course of therapy. By this time he had a degree and was working part-time to support himself. He now realized that he would need to feel successful as a man before undertaking the responsibilities of intimacy, and concentrated his energies on his career.

Both of these patients became easily disorganized by the complex tasks of intimacy. By establishing important areas of success in work, they attained levels of competence in settings that they found psychologically manageable. If they had invested themselves more strongly in intimate relationships, they might have continued to be actively symptomatic. This type of positive outcome is common in BPD. As McGlashan (1993) points out, it could be a mistake to press borderline patients too hard to become competent in sectors of their life where they have the most difficulty, rather than to capitalize on their capacities to develop competence in tasks that are less affected by their pathology.

Intermittent Treatment

The development of competence is an indicator that regular treatment can be interrupted and that the patient can be invited to try things on her or his own. Several vignettes have described the pattern in which borderline patients move in and out of treatment over an extended period. Intermittent treatment is not necessarily a problem. It may, in fact, represent for some patients a creative solution to their dilemmas in handling intimacy and attachment. Patients in supportive follow-up and multiple crisis interventions are typically seen intermittently. Many patients in intensive psychotherapies can leave treatment when they have achieved external competence, either in an intimate relationship or at work.

The following example demonstrates how different the tasks of therapy can be with the same patient at different developmental stages. The patient is the same one as described in Vignette 4.

Vignette 13

The patient had been in intensive psychotherapy from the age of 16 to 19. She made impressive gains during this time, shedding both her suicidality and her psychotic symptomatology. Her characterological impulsivity expressed itself in less destructive ways. One example was the manner in which she terminated her therapy. She had started a relationship with a new boyfriend and left treatment angrily when the therapist wanted to explore its dynamics. The explanation could be that she felt ready for more autonomy but could not work through a termination. She maintained contact over the coming years. By age 25 she had entirely recovered from BPD. At that point she was working and had a stable marriage.

At the age of 31 she returned for further treatment, which lasted for 18 months. By that time she had two young daughters and was concerned that she could damage them as her mother had damaged her. If anything, she functioned as a "supermother" whose main failing was her constant fear of disaster. Her own mother, who was still actively alcoholic, was back in her life. Most of the therapeutic work consisted of helping the patient to establish better boundaries in that relationship. In doing so, she felt more separate from her mother's pathology and less anxious about her management of her own family.

This case shows that when patients leave therapy, even impulsively, the outcome need not be negative. This patient had stopped treatment in order to attain competence in her own way, and, as it turned out, she did not need more help until she faced new adult developmental issues.

In the following case, in contrast, the passage of time failed to reduce the intensity of borderline pathology.

Vignette 14

A chronically unemployed man had first presented to an outpatient clinic with suicidal ideation at the age of 38. He had a long history of impulsive actions, including manipulative suicidal threats, substance abuse, and threats of violence to others. His marriage had ended in divorce, and his children were both troubled. He had an aggressive and outrageous manner that made him frightening to both professional staff and clinic administrative personnel. Over the years he was managed with multiple crisis interventions.

At the age of 49 he presented with a new and troubling problem. He was living with a separated woman and her 12-year-old daughter and faced a court appearance for his incestuous relationship with the child. At his reevaluation he still met all the criteria for BPD. Although he was advised by his lawyer to seek psychiatric contact, he also wanted to understand how he had gotten into this situation. He experienced the crisis as a repetition of an incident in his childhood where he had been sexually abused by an older man. He had been blamed by his parents then, and he felt he was being blamed again. To address these issues, short-term psychotherapy was prescribed, which provided him symptomatic relief.

This example shows that in some cases the treatment of BPD can be as chronic as the disorder itself. However, it is unlikely that a patient as disturbed as this could have benefited from more intensive psychotherapy, or that he could ever achieve a much higher level of competence in his life. Management by multiple crisis intervention was cost-effective, because its goal of symptomatic relief could readily be achieved.

Conclusions

The case examples in this chapter describe a range of treatment outcomes for borderline patients, from complete recovery to chronic disability. As discussed in Chapter 7, the outcome of BPD is not very predictable. The guidelines recommended here, which use the constructs of ego strength and competence, are rough measures that can at least sift out the most treatable and least treatable cases. However, outcomes for individual patients within these large groupings will offer many surprises. Some patients will have to be offered trials of therapy. In doing so, the development of a strong working alliance should be the best indicator that it is worthwhile to proceed.

Many of the vignettes demonstrate that even patients with severe borderline pathology can do well if they establish a strong alliance in the context of which they can achieve symptom control. If they have good ego strength before treatment, there is a reasonable chance they will establish at least one area of competence in their lives by the end of treatment. However, most BPD patients will continue to show some degree of emotional fragility and will need intermittent follow-up after termination.

There remain many unanswered questions about the clinical management of BPD. The need for research on treatment is one of the areas discussed in our final chapter, in which we focus on future research directions in the understanding of BPD.

Research Directions

his book is an attempt to understand borderline personality disorder in a new way. Naturally, it has raised more questions than answers. A theory of the etiology of BPD has been proposed that requires systematic investigation. Recommendations have been made for the management of borderline patients that need to be tested by clinical trials. The purpose of this last chapter is to review briefly the issues that have been discussed elsewhere in the book and to suggest what directions future investigations could take. For each of the main areas of inquiry in the previous chapters, we focus on unsolved problems and how research could shed light on them.

Definition and Boundaries

Borderline personality disorder is a misnomer, but a useful category. It describes a group of patients who have a characteristic course and who present specific and unusually challenging problems in treatment. However, the present criteria for the diagnosis of BPD are heterogeneous and lack theoretical coherence. BPD does not yet meet standard criteria for validity as a diagnostic category, in particular because of the lack of biological findings specific to the disorder.

Only a better understanding of the etiological factors in BPD will lead to a more precise definition. In the meantime, the present criteria need to be examined to determine their sensitivity and specificity. If the evidence supports doing so, the criteria should be differentially weighted to approximate more closely the prototypes used by clinicians, and hierarchical rules could be introduced to minimize any artifactual overlap of the Axis II categories. The BPD construct needs to be fine-tuned, not discarded.

The Dimensions of Borderline Personality Disorder

The dimensional approach to personality identifies underlying traits that are present prior to the development of overt disorders. Cluster analytic studies of the symptoms of BPD suggest that there are two "core dimensions" of personality that account for most of the clinical phenomenology of BPD: impulsivity and affective instability. These traits have an important theoretical link to biological theories of the personality disorders, and further studies could confirm their hypothesized relationship with the activity of neurotransmitter systems.

Identification of the dimensions of BPD could help to define a more valid disorder characterized by specific biological vulnerabilities. But it would be unwise to replace a category as clinically useful as BPD with dimensional scores. Both categorical diagnoses and dimensional measures should be used as dependent variables in future research.

Biological Risk Factors

Personality traits have a strong genetic component that is expressed in temperament. There is some evidence that the dimensions of personality have consistent associations with biological markers related to neurotransmitter systems. Thus far, no specific markers for the disorder itself have been found. There are several lines of evidence suggesting that the biological basis of BPD lies in its core dimensions.

Although future technologies may elicit more markers for BPD, most of these markers will probably continue to be related to traits. On the level of disorders, risk factors are likely, in any case, to be polygenetic. Therefore, trait markers will only have a statistical rather than a specific relation to BPD. Nevertheless, such markers could be helpful in studying the interactions of biological vulnerability with all the other risk factors for the disorder.

Psychological Risk Factors

There is evidence for a number of psychological risk factors in BPD, including trauma, neglect, and abnormal parenting. However, none of these appear to be very specific to the disorder. There may be groups of borderline patients for whom different risk factors have greater weightings, as in the subgroup who have suffered severe childhood sexual abuse. Because researchers have not examined all possible measures of childhood experience and family dysfunction, it is conceivable that there are psychological risk factors for BPD that have not yet been identified. It is also possible that some of the risk factors may have a stronger influence on specific dimensions or symptoms rather than on the overall diagnosis of BPD.

A major methodological limitation of research on psychological factors in BPD has been the use of retrospective designs. Ideally, large cohorts of children with detailed individual and family assessments should be followed prospectively for 20 years. Unfortunately, such a project would be expensive and difficult to fund. Alternatively, one could search for borderline patients among the cohorts of existing longitudinal studies. The baseline measures would have been chosen for a different purpose and would therefore not be ideal for the purpose of predicting the development of a personality disorder. Nevertheless, this method has the advantage that we would not have to risk attrition of the sample or to wait for subjects to reach maturity. The disadvantage would be that if BPD affects 1% to 2% of the population, even a cohort of 1,000 normal subjects would provide only 10 to 20 borderline patients.

Another possibility, as suggested by Gunderson and Zanarini (1989), is to study high-risk populations. A larger percentage of these populations will develop BPD, making research more practical. For example, longitudinal follow-ups of abused and neglected children could be carried out. Prospective studies would help to answer the crucial question as to why some individuals with risk factors develop severe psychopathology and others do not.

Social Risk Factors

Social risk factors in BPD could be identified from differences in prevalence of the disorder in different social classes, in cohorts over time, and in different ethnic groups or societies. To examine these issues, we need instruments to conduct epidemiological studies of BPD in the community. Given that the Diagnostic Interview Schedule used in the Epidemiologic Catchment Area study (L. N. Robins and Regier 1991) included criteria for antisocial personality disorder, it should not be that difficult to develop an instrument for this purpose.

The hypothesis offered in this book is that there is a relationship between social disintegration and BPD, and that this relationship could be demonstrated by differences in the prevalence of the disorder. A reliable measure of social disintegration would have to be developed, but could be derived from earlier research (Leighton et al. 1963). These measures should be examined for their relationship to the underlying personality dimensions of BPD, particularly impulsivity.

Multidimensional Studies

The basic theoretical position of this book is that BPD is best understood in a biopsychosocial model. The evidence thus far could support a neo-Kraepelinian version of the model, in which biological vulnerability explains the specificity of borderline pathology. These biological factors are reflected in temperamental variations, which develop in interaction with environmental factors into personality traits. These traits would then be amplified into personality disorders by psychosocial risk factors.

To test this biopsychosocial model of BPD, studies need to be carried out in which biological markers, psychological experiences, and social influences could be assessed in the same patients. These studies could then determine the relative weight of these risk factors and their

interactions with each other. This approach might also be able to identify subgroups of borderline patients who have unique weighting of the
various factors. Finally, the risk factors would be examined for their
capacity to predict both the categorical diagnosis of BPD and measures
of the core dimensions.

To carry out such an ambitious research program, we would need to
have better measures of all the risk factors. Biological measures would
have to be developed that reflect the underlying traits present in most
patients with BPD. The psychological measures would have to be well-
validated measures of childhood experience that describe a wider range
of phenomena and that have been shown to be predictors of BPD in
prospective studies. Finally, we would need valid measures of the social
risk factors for BPD.

In understanding the direction of such multidimensional research, it
is worth reconsidering the analogy, suggested in the introduction to this
book, with arteriosclerotic heart disease. Studies of the risk for myocardial infarction, such as the Framingham study (Dawber et al. 1951),
used methodologies involving longitudinal follow-up and multiple measures on large populations. It was only through these prospective and
multidimensional studies that the risk factors for coronary artery disease
were clearly identified.

Multidimensional research can be quite expensive. The more factors
that are studied, the larger the number of subjects required and the more
sites that may be needed. To make such projects possible, a number of
prerequisite conditions would have to be met. First, it would need to be
shown convincingly that BPD is a valid entity. Second, it should be well
established that BPD is associated in case-control designs with demonstrable risk factors. Finally, the increasing prevalence of BPD needs to
be documented. If BPD can be shown to be a major public health
problem, it will obtain a higher priority for research.

Outcome Research

Borderline patients get better with time, even if they never entirely
overcome their psychological fragility. The most important unanswered

question is what accounts for the variability in the outcome of BPD. We do not have good predictors of long-term outcome, but either biological, psychological, or social factors could be involved. Most of the possibilities have not been systematically examined. We need prospective studies in which many factors can be measured accurately at baseline so that groups with a better or a worse prognosis can be identified. It would be of particular clinical importance to understand why 10% of borderline patients commit suicide and 90% do not.

Another issue of clinical relevance is what happens to former borderline patients in old age. The 15-year follow-up time brings most cases into middle age. But if there is a population of formerly borderline individuals who are susceptible to further breakdown with age, or a group of cases who continue to meet BPD criteria, BPD will be of greater interest to geriatric psychiatrists.

It would also be important to understand the mechanism of improvement in BPD over time. This question could be examined in prospective studies by examining which factors best correlate with the decline of symptoms in BPD, as well as with changes in the core dimensions of the disorder.

Treatment

Treatment is the least well understood aspect of BPD. Borderline patients have a reputation for being resistant to therapy. Is this because they are untreatable, or because we have not known how to treat them? Empirical studies are just beginning to appear that measure the effectiveness of the various modalities that have been used in the treatment of BPD.

For every treatment option reviewed in Chapter 8, we need more clinical trials. Psychopharmacological interventions have been shown to be marginally valuable in treating borderline patients. The psychotherapies have received much less investigation. An important exception is the recent research on the effectiveness of cognitive-behavior therapy in borderline patients (Linehan et al. 1991), but we need to know whether these effects are stable over time.

Identifying the mechanism for naturalistic improvement in borderline patients could be useful in determining the direction of treatment. For example, if the decline of impulsivity is crucial to improvement in BPD, treatments should be targeted for this dimension.

Because the theory behind an intervention and its actual mechanism of action could be entirely different, studies are needed that separate specific from nonspecific effects in the therapy of BPD. The best method would be to carry out comparative studies between modalities that involve the same level of time and input. Studies that measure the outcome of complex treatment methods are also needed to sort out which interventions are the most effective. Finally, there may be important subgroups of borderline patients who respond to different treatment approaches.

Some of these questions could be answered by large-scale projects that examine the treatment of BPD over long periods of time. In view of the chronicity of borderline psychopathology, long-term follow-up of treated patients is necessary to assess the stability of change. We know from research on other chronic conditions, such as eating disorders (Bruch 1978), that short-term improvement can be highly misleading when relapse is the rule.

Longitudinal studies of borderline patients in treatment would also make it possible to test some of the hypotheses about clinical management presented in Chapter 9. Such research could provide a more rational basis for the triage and management of BPD, but would require a large cohort of patients. Measures of ego strength and of work history could be used as short-term predictors of therapeutic alliance formation and as long-term predictors of outcome. It is also possible the subgroups of more or less treatable patients could be identified by dimensional measures of personality. In a large-scale study, one could also test hypotheses about the matching of subgroups of borderline patients to different treatment modalities.

Conclusion

It would be worthwhile at this point to review the main themes of this book. The first is that the etiology of mental disorders in general, and of personality disorders in particular, depends on an amalgam of many risk factors. It is for this reason that biopsychosocial models are needed to understand these factors. Disorders with multiple etiological factors also require multidimensional treatment that makes use of a wide armamentarium of interventions. There will never be a simple explanation for the etiology, course, or treatment response of BPD.

The second theme of this book has been that future progress in understanding BPD can only come from empirical research. Psychodynamic understanding is relevant to individual cases but does not explain phenomena that are common to borderline patients as a group. To the extent that BPD is a valid diagnosis, it describes a category of patients who present with characteristic clinical features and clinical problems. To understand these commonalities requires scientific methods.

It is worth reiterating that the emphasis on scientific psychiatry in this book need not be associated with a reductionistic point of view. Multidimensional research on mental disorders, including borderline personality disorder, has the capacity to take into account the complex phenomena of the real world. It is precisely this complexity that accounts for the endless fascination of psychiatry.

References

Aarkrog T: Borderline adolescents 20 years later. Paper presented to the International Society for the Study of Personality Disorders, Cambridge, MA, September 1993

Adler G: The myth of the alliance in borderline patients. Am J Psychiatry 136:642–645, 1979

Adler G: Borderline Psychopathology and Its Treatment. New York, Jason Aronson, 1985

Akiskal HS: Depression in the historical perspective. Paper presented at the 144th annual meeting of the American Psychiatric Association, New Orleans, LA, May 1991

Akiskal HS, Chen SE, Davis GC, et al: Borderline: an adjective in search of a noun. J Clin Psychiatry 46:41–48, 1985

Alexander F, French T: Psychoanalytic Therapy. New York, Ronald Press, 1946

American Psychiatric Association: Diagnostic and Statistical Manual of Mental Disorders. Washington, DC, American Psychiatric Association, 1952

American Psychiatric Association: Diagnostic and Statistical Manual of Mental Disorders, 2nd Edition. Washington, DC, American Psychiatric Association, 1968

American Psychiatric Association: Diagnostic and Statistical Manual of Mental Disorders, 3rd Edition. Washington, DC, American Psychiatric Association, 1980

American Psychiatric Association: Diagnostic and Statistical Manual of Mental Disorders, 3rd Edition, Revised. Washington, DC, American Psychiatric Association, 1987

American Psychiatric Association: Diagnostic and Statistical Manual of Mental Disorders, 4th Edition. Washington, DC, American Psychiatric Association, 1994

Andrulonis PA, Glueck BC, Stroebel CF, et al: Borderline personality subcategories. J Nerv Ment Dis 170:670–679, 1982

Anthony EJ, Cohler BJ (eds): The Invulnerable Child. New York, Guilford, 1987

Aronson TA: A critical review of psychotherapeutic treatments of the borderline personality. J Nerv Ment Dis 177:511–528, 1989

Åsberg M, Träskman L, Thorén P: 5-HIAA in the cerebrospinal fluid: a biochemical suicide predictor? Arch Gen Psychiatry 33:1193–1197, 1976

Bandura A: Social Learning Theory. Englewood Cliffs, NJ, Prentice-Hall, 1977

Bardenstein KK, McGlashan TH: The natural history of a residentially treated borderline sample: gender differences. Journal of Personality Disorders 3:69–83, 1989

Barlow DH: Anxiety and Its Disorders: The Nature and Treatment of Anxiety and Panic. New York, Guilford, 1988

Baron M, Gruen R, Asnis L, et al: Familial transmission of schizotypal and borderline personality disorders. Am J Psychiatry 142:927–934, 1985

Beavers WR: Psychotherapy and Growth: A Family Systems Perspective. New York, Brunner/Mazel, 1977

Beck AT, Freeman A: Cognitive Therapy of Personality Disorders. New York, Guilford, 1990

Belsky J, Steinberg L, Draper P: Childhood experience, interpersonal development, and reproductive: an evolutionary theory of socialization. Child Dev 62:647–670, 1991

Benedict R: Patterns of Culture. New York, Houghton-Mifflin, 1961

Benjamin LS: An interpersonal approach to the diagnosis of borderline personality disorder, in Borderline Personality Disorder: Clinical and Empirical Perspectives. Edited by Clarkin JF, Marziali E, Munroe-Blum H. New York, Guilford, 1992, pp 161–196

Bernstein EM, Putnam FW: Development, reliability, and validity of a dissociation scale. J Nerv Ment Dis 174:727–735, 1986

Bezirganian S, Cohen P, Brook JS: The impact of mother-child interaction on the development of borderline personality disorder. Am J Psychiatry 150:1836–1842, 1993

Blackwell B: Newer antidepressant drugs, in Psychopharmacology: The Third Generation of Progress. Edited by Meltzer HY. New York, Raven, 1987, pp 1041–1049

Blashfield R: The Classification of Psychopathology: Neo-Kraepelinian and Quantitative Approaches. New York, Plenum, 1984

Blashfield R, Blum N, Pfohl B: The effects of changing Axis II diagnostic criteria. Compr Psychiatry 33:245–252, 1992

Blashfield R, Herkov MJ: Hierarchy of DSM-III-R personality disorders, in New Research Program and Abstracts, 146th annual meeting of the American Psychiatric Association, San Francisco, CA, May 1993, NR507, p 187

Bleuler E: Dementia Praecox or the Group of Schizophrenias (1911). Translated by Zinkin J. New York, International Universities Press, 1950

Bond M, Gardner ST, Christian J, et al: Empirical study of self-rated defense styles. Arch Gen Psychiatry 40:333–338, 1983

Bond M: Are "borderline defenses" specific to borderline personality disorder? Journal of Personality Disorders 4:251–256, 1990

Bond M, Paris J, Zweig-Frank H: The Defense Style Questionnaire in borderline personality disorder. Journal of Personality Disorders 8:28–31, 1994

Bouchard TJ, Lykken DT, McGue M, et al: Sources of human psychological differences: the Minnesota study of twins reared apart. Science 250:223–228, 1990

Bowlby J: Attachment and Loss, Vol 1: Attachment. London, Hogarth Press, 1969

Bowlby J: Attachment and Loss, Vol 2: Separation: Anxiety and Anger. London, Hogarth Press, 1973

Bowlby J: Attachment and Loss, Vol 3: Loss: Sadness and Depression. London, Hogarth Press, 1980

Bradley SJ: The relationship of early maternal separation to borderline personality in children and adolescents: a pilot study. Am J Psychiatry 136:424–426, 1979

Brewin CR, Andrews B, Gotlib IH: Psychopathology and early experience: a reappraisal of retrospective reports. Psychol Bull 113:82–98, 1993

Briere J, Zaidi LY: Sexual abuse histories and sequelae in female psychiatric emergency room patients, Am J Psychiatry 146:1602–1606, 1989

Brown GL, Goodwin FK, Ballenger JC, et al: Aggression in humans correlates with cerebrospinal fluid amine metabolites. Psychiatry Res 1:131–139, 1979

Brown GR, Anderson B: Psychiatric morbidity in adult inpatients with childhood histories of sexual and physical abuse. Am J Psychiatry 148:55–61, 1991

Browne A, Finkelhor D: Impact of child sexual abuse: a review of the literature. Psychol Bull 99:66–77, 1986

Bruch H: The Golden Cage, the Enigma of Anorexia Nervosa. Cambridge, MA, Harvard University Press, 1978

Buchsbaum MS: Average evoked response and stimulus intensity in identical and fraternal twins. Physiol Psychol 2:365–370, 1974

Burgess RL, Conger PD: Family interaction in abusive, neglectful and normal families. Child Dev 49:1163–1173, 1978

Buss DM, Plomin R: Temperament: Early Developing Personality Traits. Hillsdale, NJ, Lawrence Erlbaum, 1984

Byrne CP, Velamoor VR, Cernovsky ZZ, et al: A comparison of borderline and schizophrenic patients for childhood life events and parent-child relationships. Can J Psychiatry 35:590–595, 1990

Carpenter WT Jr, Gunderson JG, Strauss JS: Considerations of the borderline syndrome: a longitudinal comparative study of borderline and schizophrenic patients, in Borderline Personality Disorders: The Concept, the Syndrome, the Patient. Edited by Hartocollis P. New York, International Universities Press, 1977, pp 223–254

Chess S, Thomas A: Origins and Evolution of Behavior Disorders: From Infancy to Early Adult Life. New York, Brunner/Mazel, 1984

Chess S, Thomas A: The New York Longitudinal Study (NYLS): the young adult periods. Can J Psychiatry 35:557–561, 1990

Chu JA, Dill DL: Dissociative symptoms in relation to childhood physical and sexual abuse. Am J Psychiatry 147:887–892, 1990

Clarke A, Clarke A: Early Experience and Behavior. New York, Free Press, 1979

Clarkin JF, Kernberg OF: Developmental factors in borderline personality disorder and borderline personality organization, in Borderline Personality Disorder: Etiology and Treatment. Edited by Paris J. Washington, DC, American Psychiatric Press, 1993, pp 161–184

Clarkin JF, Widiger TA, Frances A, et al: Propotypic typology and the borderline personality disorder. J Abnorm Psychol 92:263–275, 1983

Clarkin JF, Koenigsberg H, Yeomans F, et al: Psychodynamic psychotherapy of the borderline patient, in Borderline Personality Disorder: Clinical and Empirical Perspectives. Edited by Clarkin JF, Marziali E, Munroe-Blum H. New York, Guilford, 1992, pp 268–287

Clarkin JF, Hull JW, Cantor J, et al: Borderline personality disorder and personality traits: a comparison of SCID-II BPD and NEO-PI. Psychological Assessment 5:472–476, 1993

Cloninger CR: A systematic method for clinical description and classification of personality variants: a proposal. Arch Gen Psychiatry 44:573–588, 1987

Cloninger CR: Structure and inheritance of personality dimensions. Paper presented to the Second International Congress on the Disorders of the Personality. Oslo, Norway, July 1991

Cloninger CR, Dinwiddie SH, Reich T: Epidemiology and genetics of alcoholism, in American Psychiatric Press Review of Psychiatry, Vol 8. Edited by Tasman A, Hales RE, Frances AJ. Washington, DC, American Psychiatric Press, 1989, pp 293–308

Cloninger CR, Martin RL, Guze SB, et al: The empirical structure of psychiatric comorbidity and its theoretical significance, in Comorbidity of Mood and Anxiety Disorders. Edited by Maser JD, Cloninger CR. Washington, DC, American Psychiatric Press, 1990, pp 439–462

Cloninger CR, Svrakic DM, Przybeck TR:: A psychobiological model of temperament and character. Arch Gen Psychiatry 50:975–990, 1993

Coccaro EF: Biological validators of personality disorders. Paper presented at the 144th annual meeting of the American Psychiatric Association, New Orleans, LA, May 1991

Coccaro EF, Siever LJ, Klar HM, et al: Serotonergic studies in patients with affective and personality disorders: correlates with suicidal and impulsive aggressive behavior. Arch Gen Psychiatry 46:587–599, 1989

Committee on Sexual Offences Against Children and Youth, Canada [Badgley RF, chairman]: Sexual Offence Against Children. Ottawa, Supply and Services Canada, 1984

Conte JR, Wolf S, Smith T: What sexual offenders tell us about prevention strategies. Child Abuse Negl 13:293–301, 1989

Cornelius JR, Soloff PH, Perel JM, et al: Fluoxetine trial in borderline personality disorder. Psychopharmacol Bull 26:151–154, 1990

Cornelius JR, Soloff PH, Perel JM, et al: Continuation pharmacotherapy of borderline personality disorder with haloperidol and phenelzine. Am J Psychiatry 150:1843–1848, 1993

Costa PT Jr, McCrae RR: From catalog to classification: Murray's needs and the five-factor model. J Pers Soc Psychol 55:258–265, 1988

Costa PT Jr, Widiger TA: Personality Disorders and the Five-Factor Model of Personality. Washington, DC, American Psychological Association, 1994

Courtois CA: Healing the Incest Wound: Adult Survivors in Therapy. New York, WW Norton, 1988

Cowdry RW, Gardner DL: Pharmacotherapy of borderline personality disorder: alprazolam, carbamazepine, trifluoperazine, and tranylcypromine. Arch Gen Psychiatry 45:111–119, 1988

Dawber TR, Meadors GF, Moore FE: Epidemiological approaches to heart disease: the Framingham study. Am J Publ Health 41:279–286, 1951

Dawson DF: Treatment of the borderline patient, relationship management. Can J Psychiatry 33:370–374, 1988

Dawson DF, MacMillan HL: Relationship Management of the Borderline Patient: From Understanding to Treatment. New York, Brunner/Mazel, 1993

Deutsch A: Observations on a sidewalk ashram. Arch Gen Psychiatry 32:166–175, 1975

DiNicola VF: Family therapy and transcultural psychiatry, an emerging synthesis. Transcultural Psychiatric Research Review 22:151–180, 1985

DiNicola VF: Anorexia multiforme: self-starvation in historical and cultural context. Transcultural Psychiatric Research Review 27:165–196, 1990

Dohrenwend BP, Dohrenwend BS, Gould MS, et al: Mental Illness in the United States: Epidemiological Estimates. New York, Praeger, 1980

Drake RE, Gates C, Cotton PG, et al: Suicide among schizophrenics: who is at risk? J Nerv Ment Dis 172:613–617, 1984

Dunn J, Plomin R: Separate Lives: Why Siblings Are So Different. New York, Basic Books, 1990

Dupré J (ed): The Latest on the Best. Cambridge, MA, MIT Press, 1987

Durkheim E: Suicide: A Study in Sociology (1897). Translated by Spaulding JA, Simpson G. Edited by Simpson G. New York, Free Press, 1951

Eaton WW: The Sociology of Mental Disorders. New York, Praeger, 1986

Endicott J, Spitzer RL, Fleiss JL, et al: The Global Assessment Scale: a procedure for measuring overall severity of psychiatric disturbance. Arch Gen Psychiatry 33:766–771, 1976

Engel GL: The clinical application of the biopsychosocial model. Am J Psychiatry 137:535–544, 1980

Erikson EH: Childhood and Society. New York, WW Norton, 1950

Eysenck HJ: Culture and personality abnormalities, in Culture and Psychopathology. Edited by Al-Issa I. Baltimore, MD, University Park Press, 1982, pp 277–308

Eysenck HJ: Biological dimensions of personality, in Handbook of Personality: Theory and Research. Edited by Pervin LA. New York, Guilford, 1990, pp 244–276

Eysenck HJ: Genetic and environmental contributions to individual differences: the three major dimensions of personality. J Pers 58:245–261, 1991

Fabrega H Jr, Ulrich R, Pilkonis P, et al: On the homogeneity of personality disorder clusters. Compr Psychiatry 32:373–386, 1991

Fava M, Rosenbaum JF: Suicidality and fluoxetine: is there a relationship? J Clin Psychiatry 52:108–111, 1991

Feighner JP, Robins E, Guze SB, et al: Diagnostic criteria for use in psychiatric research. Arch Gen Psychiatry 26:57–63, 1972

Feldman RB, Guttman HA: Families of borderline patients: literal-minded parents, borderline parents, and parental protectiveness. Am J Psychiatry 141:1392–1396, 1984

Finkelhor D: A Sourcebook on Child Sexual Abuse. Beverly Hills, CA, Sage, 1986

Finkelhor D: The trauma of child sexual abuse: two models, in Lasting Effects of Child Sexual Abuse. Edited by Wyatt GE, Powell GJ. Beverly Hills, CA, Sage, 1988, pp 61–82

Finkelhor D, Hotaling G, Lewis IA, et al: Sexual abuse in a national survey of adult men and women: prevalence characteristics and risk factors. Child Abuse Negl 14:19–28, 1990

Flavin DK, Franklin JE Jr, Frances RJ: Substance abuse and suicidal behavior, in Suicide Over the Life Cycle: Risk Factors, Assessment, and Treatment of Suicidal Patients. Edited by Blumenthal SJ, Kupfer DJ. Washington, DC, American Psychiatric Press, 1990, pp 177–204

Frances AJ, Widiger T: The classification of personality disorders: an overview of problems and solutions. Psychiatry Update: American Psychiatric Association Annual Review, Vol 5. Edited by Frances AJ, Hales RE. Washington, DC, American Psychiatric Press, 1986, pp 240–257

Frances A[J], Clarkin J[F], Perry S: Differential Therapeutics in Psychiatry: The Art and Science of Treatment Selection. New York, Brunner/Mazel, 1984

Frank AF: The therapeutic alliances of borderline patients, in Borderline Personality Disorder: Clinical and Empirical Perspectives. Edited by Clarkin JF, Marziali E, Munroe-Blum H. New York, Guilford, 1992, pp 220–247

Frank H, Paris J: Recollections of family experience in borderline patients. Arch Gen Psychiatry 38:1031–1034, 1981

Friedman HJ: Psychotherapy of borderline patients: the influence of theory on technique. Am J Psychiatry 132:1048–1052, 1975

Friedman HJ: Review: Waldinger RJ and Gunderson JG, Effective psychotherapy with borderline patients: case studies. Am J Psychiatry 146:1336–1337, 1989

Friis S: A personal follow-up of patients with personality disorders treated in a day unit. Paper presented to the International Society for the Study of Personality Disorders, Cambridge, MA, September 1993

Fromuth ME: The relationship of childhood sexual abuse with later psychological and sexual adjustment in a sample of college women. Child Abuse Negl 10:5–15, 1986

Gardner DL, Cowdry RW: Positive effects of carbamazepine on behavioral dyscontrol in borderline personality disorder. Am J Psychiatry 143:519–522, 1986

Gardner DL, Lucas PB, Cowdry RW: CSF metabolites in borderline personality disorder compared with normal controls. Biol Psychiatry 28:247–254, 1990

Gardner H: Frames of Mind: The Theory of Multiple Intelligences. New York, Basic Books, 1977

Garfield SL: Research on client variables in psychotherapy, in Handbook of Psychotherapy and Behavior Change, 3rd Edition. Edited by Garfield SL, Bergin AE. New York, Wiley, 1986, pp 213–256

Garfield SL, Bergin AE: Handbook of Psychotherapy and Behavior Change, 3rd Edition. New York, Wiley, 1986

Garmezy N, Rutter M (eds): Stress, Coping and Development in Children. New York, McGraw-Hill, 1983

Glick ID, Hargreaves WA, Drues J, et al: Short vs long hospitalization: a prospective controlled study, VII: two-year follow-up results for nonschizophrenics. Arch Gen Psychiatry 34:314–317, 1977

Goldberg RL, Mann LS, Sie TN: Parental qualities as perceived by borderline personality disorders. Hillside J Clin Psychiatry 7:134–140, 1985

Goldberg SC, Schulz SC, Schulz PM, et al: Borderline and schizotypal personality disorders treated with low-dose thiothixene vs placebo. Arch Gen Psychiatry 43:680–686, 1986

Gordon RA: Anorexia and Bulemia. Cambridge, UK, Blackwell Scientific, 1990

Gottesman II: Schizophrenia Genesis: The Origins of Madness. New York, WH Freeman, 1991

Gould SJ, Lewontin RC: The spandrels of San Marco and the Panglossian paradigm: a critique of the adaptationist programme. Proc Royal Soc London 205:581–598, 1979

Goyer PF, Andreason PJ, Semple WE, et al: PET and personality disorders. Paper presented to the Second International Congress on the Disorders of the Personality, Oslo, Norway, July 1991

Gunderson JG: Borderline Personality Disorder. Washington, DC, American Psychiatric Press, 1984

Gunderson JG, Kolb JE: Discriminating features of borderline patients. Am J Psychiatry 135:792–796, 1978

Gunderson JG, Phillips KA: A current view of the interface between borderline personality disorder and depression. Am J Psychiatry 148:967–975, 1991

Gunderson JG, Pollack WS: Conceptual risks of the Axis I–II division, in Biologic Response Styles: Clinical Implications. Edited by Klar H, Siever LJ. Washington, DC, American Psychiatric Press, 1985, pp 81–95

Gunderson JG, Sabo AN: The phenomenological and conceptual interface between borderline personality disorder and PTSD. Am J Psychiatry 150:19–27, 1993

Gunderson JG, Singer MT: Defining borderline patients: an overview. Am J Psychiatry 132:1–10, 1975

Gunderson JG, Zanarini MC: Pathogenesis of borderline personality, in American Psychiatric Press Review of Psychiatry, Vol 8. Edited by Tasman A, Hales RE, Frances AJ. Washington, DC, American Psychiatric Press, 1989, pp 25–48

Gunderson JG, Kerr J, Englund DW: The families of borderlines: a comparative study. Arch Gen Psychiatry 37:27–33, 1980

Gunderson JG, Frank AF, Ronningstam EF, et al: Early discontinuance of borderline patients from psychotherapy. J Nerv Ment Dis 177:38–42, 1989

Gunderson JG, Zanarini MC, Kisiel CL: Borderline personality disorder: a review of data on DSM-III-R descriptions. Journal of Personality Disorders 5:340–352, 1991

Gurrera RJ: Some biological and behavioral features associated with clinical personality types. J Nerv Ment Dis 178:556–566, 1990

Guze SB, Robins E: Suicide and primary affective disorders. Br J Psychiatry 117:437–438, 1970

Harding CM, Brooks GW, Ashikaga T, et al: The Vermont Longitudinal Study of Persons With Severe Mental Illness, I: methodology, study sample, and overall status 32 years later. Am J Psychiatry 144:718–726, 1987a

Harding CM, Brooks GW, Ashikaga T, et al: The Vermont Longitudinal Study of Persons With Severe Mental Illness, II: long-term outcome of subjects who retrospectively met DSM-III criteria for schizophrenia. Am J Psychiatry 144:727–735, 1987b

Herman JL: Trauma and Recovery. New York, Basic Books, 1992

Herman JL, Schatzow E: Recovery and verification of memories of childhood sexual trauma. Psychoanalytic Psychology 4:11–14, 1987

Herman JL, van der Kolk B: Traumatic antecedents of borderline personality disorder, in Psychological Trauma. Edited by van der Kolk BA. Washington, DC, American Psychiatric Press, 1987, pp 111–126

Herman JL, Perry JC, van der Kolk BA: Childhood trauma in borderline personality disorder. Am J Psychiatry 146:490–495, 1989

Hoch PH, Cattell JP, Strahl MO, et al: The course and outcome of pseudoneurotic schizophrenia. Am J Psychiatry 119:106–115, 1962

Hogarty GE, Schooler NR, Ulrich R, et al: Fluphenazine and social therapy in the aftercare of schiozphrenic patients: relapse analyses of a two-year controlled study of fluphenazine decanoate and fluphenazine hydrochloride. Arch Gen Psychiatry 36:1283–1294, 1979

Horowitz MJ: Stress Response Syndromes. New York, Jason Aronson, 1976

Horwitz L: Clinical Prediction in Psychotherapy. New York, Jason Aronson, 1974

Hurt SW, Clarkin JF, Munroe-Blum H, et al: Borderline behavioral clusters and different treatment approaches, in Borderline Personality Disorder: Clinical and Empirical Perspectives. Edited by Clarkin JF, Marziali E, Munroe-Blum H. New York, Guilford, 1992, pp 199–219

Inkeles A, Smith DH: Becoming Modern: Individual Change in Six Developing Countries. Cambridge, MA, Harvard University Press, 1974

Jason J, Williams SL, Burton A, et al: Epidemiological differences between sexual and physical abuse. JAMA 247:3344–3348, 1982

Jilek-Aall L: Suicidal behavior among youth: a cross-cultural comparison. Transcultural Psychiatric Research Review 25:87–105, 1988

Kagan J: The Nature of the Child. New York, Basic Books, 1984

Kagan J: Shyness and personality disorders. Paper presented to the International Society for the Study of Personality Disorders, Cambridge, MA, September 1993

Kagan J, Resnick JS, Snidman N, et al: Childhood derivatives of inhibition and lack of inhibition to the unfamiliar. Child Dev 59:1580–1589, 1988

Kauffman C, Grunebaum H, Cohler B, et al: Superkids: competent children of psychotic mothers. Am J Psychiatry 136:1398–1402, 1979

Kelley WE (ed): Post-Traumatic Stress Disorder and the War Veteran Patient. New York, Brunner/Mazel, 1985

Kernberg OF: Borderline Conditions and Pathological Narcissism. New York, Jason Aronson, 1975

Kernberg OF: Severe Personality Disorders: Psychotherapeutic Strategies. New Haven, CT, Yale University Press, 1984

Kernberg OF, Burstein ED, Coyne L, et al: Psychotherapy and psychoanalysis: final report of the Menninger Foundation's Psychotherapy Research Project. Bull Menninger Clin 36:1–275, 1972

Kernberg OF, Selzer MA, Koenigsberg HW, et al: Psychodynamic Psychotherapy of Borderline Patients. New York, Basic Books, 1990

Kjelsberg E, Eikeseth PH, Dahl AA: Suicide in borderline patients—predictive factors. Acta Psychiatr Scand 84:283–287, 1991

Klein DF: Psychopharmacological treatment and delineation of borderline disorders, in Borderline Personality Disorders: The Concept, the Syndrome, the Patient. Edited by Hartocollis P. New York, International Universities Press, 1977, pp 365–384

Klerman GL: Historical perspectives on contemporary schools of psychopathology, in Contemporary Directions in Psychopathology: Toward the DSM-IV. Edited by Millon T, Klerman GL. New York, Guilford, 1986, pp 3–28

Kohut H: The Analysis of the Self: A Systematic Approach to the Psychoanalytic Treatment of Narcissistic Personality Disorders. New York, International Universities Press, 1971

Kraepelin E: Dementia Praecox and Paraphrenia (1919). New York, Krieger, 1971

Kroll J: The Challenge of the Borderline Patient: Competency in Diagnosis and Treatment. New York, WW Norton, 1988

Kroll J: PTSD/Borderlines in Therapy: Finding the Balance. New York, WW Norton, 1993

Kroll J, Carey K, Sines L: Are there borderlines in Britain? A cross-validation of US findings. Arch Gen Psychiatry 39:60–63, 1982

Kuhn TA: The Structure of Scientific Revolutions, 2nd Edition. Chicago, IL, University of Chicago Press, 1970

Kullgren G: Factors associated with completed suicide in borderline personality disorder. J Nerv Ment Dis 176:40–44, 1988

Kutcher SP, Blackwood DHR, St Clair D, et al: Auditory P300 in borderline personality disorder and schizophrenia. Arch Gen Psychiatry 44:645–650, 1987

Lasch C: The Culture of Narcissism. New York, Warner Books, 1979a

Lasch C: Haven in a Heartless World: The Family Besieged. New York, Basic Books, 1979b

Lasch C: The True and Only Heaven: Progress and Its Critics. New York, Basic Books, 1991

Lazarus RS, Folkman S: Stress, Appraisal and Coping. New York, Springer, 1984

Leary T: Interpersonal Diagnosis of Personality. New York, Ronald Press, 1957

Leibenluft E, Gardner DL, Cowdry RW: The inner experience of the borderline self-mutilator. Journal of Personality Disorders 1:317–324, 1987

Leighton DC, Harding JS, Macklin DB, et al: The Character of Danger: Psychiatric Symptoms in Selected Communities. New York, Basic Books, 1963

Lesage AD, Boyer R, Grunberg F, et al: Childhood separations, Axis II and suicide. Paper presented at the 146th annual meeting of the American Psychiatric Association, San Francisco, CA, May 1993

Lesage AD, Boyer R, Grunberg F, et al: Suicide and mental disorders: a case-control study of young males. Am J Psychiatry (in press)

Levy D: Maternal Overprotection. New York, Columbia University Press, 1943

Lewis JM, Beavers WR, Gossett JT, et al (eds): No Single Thread: Psychological Health in Family Systems, New York, Brunner/Mazel, 1976

Lewontin RC: The Genetic Basis of Evolutionary Change. New York, Columbia University Press, 1974

Linehan MM: Dialectical behavior therapy for borderline personality disorder: theory and method. Bull Menninger Clin 51:261–276, 1987

Linehan MM: Cognitive Behavioral Therapy of Borderline Personality Disorder. New York, Guilford, 1993

Linehan MM, Koerner K: A behavioral theory of borderline personality disorder, in Borderline Personality Disorder: Etiology and Treatment. Edited by Paris J. Washington, DC, American Psychiatric Press, 1993, pp 103–121

Linehan MM, Armstrong HE, Suarez A, et al: Cognitive-behavioral treatment of chronically parasuicidal borderline patients. Arch Gen Psychiatry 48:1060–1064, 1991

Linehan MM, Heard HL, Armstrong HE: Naturalistic follow-up of a behavioral treatment for chronically parasuicidal borderline patients. Arch Gen Psychiatry 50:971–974, 1993

Links PS, Boiago I: N of 1 randomized control trial for BPD patients (letter). Can J Psychiatry 37:148, 1992

Links PS, Boiago I: Borderline personality disorder as an impulse disorder: evidence from family and genetic studies. Journal of Personality Disorders (in press)

Links PS, van Reekum R: Childhood sexual abuse, parental impairment and the development of borderline personality disorder. Can J Psychiatry 38:472–474, 1993

Links PS, Steiner M, Huxley G: The occurrence of borderline personality disorder in the families of borderline patients. Journal of Personality Disorders 2:14–20, 1988a

Links PS, Steiner M, Offord DR, et al: Characteristics of borderline personality disorder: a Canadian study. Can J Psychiatry 33:336–340, 1988b

Links PS, Mitton JE, Steiner M: Predicting outcome for borderline personality disorder. Compr Psychiatry 31:490–498, 1990a

Links PS, Steiner M, Boiago I, et al: Lithium therapy for borderline patients: preliminary findings. Journal of Personality Disorders 4:173–181, 1990b

Links PS, Fedorov C, Mitton J, et al: Patients who are no longer borderline. Paper presented at the 146th annual meeting of the American Psychiatric Association, San Francisco, CA, May 1993

Livesley WJ: Trait and behavioral prototypes of personality disorder. Am J Psychiatry 143:728–732, 1986

Livesley WJ, Schroeder ML: Dimensions of personality disorder: the DSM-III-R cluster B diagnoses. J Nerv Ment Dis 179:320–328, 1991

Livesley WJ, Jackson DN, Schroeder ML: A study of the factorial study of personality pathology. Journal of Personality Disorders 3:292–306, 1989

Livesley WJ, Jackson DN, Schroeder ML: Factorial structure of traits delineating personality disorders in clinical and general population samples. J Abnorm Psychol 101:432–440, 1992

Livesley WJ, Jang KL, Jackson DN, et al: Genetic and environmental contributions to dimensions of personality disorders. Am J Psychiatry 150:1826–1831, 1993

Loftus EF: The reality of repressed memories. Am Psychol 48:518–537, 1993

Loranger AW, Oldham JM, Tulis EH: Familial transmission of DSM-III borderline personality disorder. Arch Gen Psychiatry 39:795–799, 1982

Loranger AW, Hirschfeld RMA, Sartorius N, et al: The WHO/AD-AMHA International Pilot Study of Personality Disorders: background and purpose, Journal of Personality Disorders 5:296–306, 1991

Luborsky L: Clinicians' judgments of mental health: a proposed scale. Arch Gen Psychiatry 7:407–417, 1962

Luborsky L: Who Will Benefit From Psychotherapy? New York, Basic Books, 1988

Luborsky L, Singer B, Luborsky L: Comparative studies of psychotherapies: is it true that "everyone has won and all must have prizes"? Arch Gen Psychiatry 32:995–1008, 1975

Ludolph PS, Westen D, Misle B, et al: The borderline diagnosis in adolescents: symptoms and developmental history. Am J Psychiatry 147:470–476, 1990

Lykken DT, McGue M, Tellegen A, et al: Emergenesis: genetic traits that may not run in families. Am Psychol 47:1565–1577, 1992

MacDonald MJ: Speculation on the evolution of insulin-dependent diabetes genes. Metabolism 37:1182–1184, 1988

Maddocks PD: A five year follow-up of untreated psychopaths. Br J Psychiatry 116: 511–515, 1970

Main M, Kaplan N, Cassidy J: Security in infancy, childhood, and adulthood: a move to the level of representation. Monogr Soc Res Child Dev 50:66–104, 1985

Malinosky-Rummell R, Hansen DJ: Long-term consequences of physical abuse. Psychol Bull 114:68–79, 1993

Maris RW: Pathways to Suicide: A Survey of Self-Destructive Behaviors. Baltimore, MD, Johns Hopkins University Press, 1981

Maris RW, Berman AL, Maltsberger JT, et al (eds): Assessment and Prediction of Suicide. New York, Guilford, 1992

Markowitz PJ: SSRI treatment of borderline personality. Paper presented to the International Society for the Study of Personality Disorders, Cambridge, MA, September 1993

Markowitz PJ, Calabrese JR, Schulz SC, et al: Fluoxetine in borderline and schizotypal personality disorders. Paper presented at the annual meeting of the Society for Biological Psychiatry, New York, May 1990

Martial J, Paris J, Zweig-Frank H, et al: Study of serotonergic function in borderline personality disorder by the fenfluramine challenge test. Paper presented to Club des Recherches Cliniques du Quebec, September 1993

Marttunen MJ, Aro HM, Henriksson MM, et al: Mental disorders in adolescent suicide: DSM-III-R Axes I and II diagnoses in suicides among 13- to 19-year-olds in Finland. Arch Gen Psychiatry 48:834–839, 1991

Masterson JF, Rinsley DB: The borderline syndrome: the role of the mother in the genesis and psychic structure of the borderline personality. Int J Psychoanal 56:163–177, 1975

McGlashan TH: The prediction of outcome in borderline personality disorder: Part V of the Chestnut Lodge follow-up study, in The Borderline: Current Empirical Research. Edited by McGlashan TH. Washington, DC, American Psychiatric Press, 1985, pp 61–98

McGlashan TH: The Chestnut Lodge follow-up study, III: long-term outcome of borderline personalities. Arch Gen Psychiatry 43:20–30, 1986

McGlashan TH: Implications of outcome research for the treatment of borderline personality disorder, in Borderline Personality Disorder: Etiology and Treatment. Edited by Paris J. Washington, DC, American Psychiatric Press, 1993, pp 235–259

McGoldrick M, Pearce JK, Giordano J (eds): Ethnicity and Family Therapy. New York, Guilford, 1982

McGuffin P, Thapar A: The genetics of personality disorder. Br J Psychiatry 160:12–23, 1992

Mednick SA, Moffit T (eds): Biology and Crime. Cambridge, UK, Cambridge University Press, 1985

Meehl PE: Toward an integrated theory of schizotaxa, schizotypy, and schizophrenia. Journal of Personality Disorders 4:1–99, 1990

Melges FT, Swartz MS: Oscillations of attachment in borderline personality disorder. Am J Psychiatry 146:1115–1120, 1989

Millman RB: [Drug abuse and drug dependence] General principles of diagnosis and treatment, in Psychiatry Update: American Psychiatric Association Annual Review, Vol 5. Edited by Frances AJ, Hales RE. Washington, DC, American Psychiatric Press, 1986, pp 122–136

Millon T: Disorders of Personality: DSM-III Axis II. New York, Wiley, 1981

Millon T: On the genesis and prevalence of borderline personality disorder: a social learning thesis. Journal of Personality Disorders 1:354–372, 1987

Millon T: Borderline personality disorder: a psychosocial epidemic, in Borderline Personality Disorder: Etiology and Treatment. Edited by Paris J. Washington, DC, American Psychiatric Press, 1993, pp 197–210

Minuchin S: Families and Family Therapy. Cambridge, MA, Harvard University Press, 1974

Morey LC, Ochoa ES: An investigation of adherence to diagnostic criteria: clinical diagnosis of the DSM-III personality disorders. Journal of Personality Disorders 3:183–192, 1989

Munroe-Blum H: Group treatment of borderline personality disorder, in Borderline Personality Disorder: Clinical and Empirical Perspectives. Edited by Clarkin JF, Marziali E, Munroe-Blum H. New York, Guilford, 1992, pp 288–299

Murphy DL, Mellow AM, Sunderland T, et al: Strategies for the study of serotonin in humans, in Serotonin in Major Psychiatric Disorders. Edited by Coccaro EF, Murphy DL. Washington, DC, American Psychiatric Press, 1990, pp 1–25

Murphy HBM: Comparative Psychiatry. New York, Springer-Verlag, 1982

Nash MR, Hulsey TL, Sexton MC, et al: Long-term sequelae of childhood sexual abuse: perceived family environment, psychopathology, and dissociation. J Consult Clin Psychol 61:276–283, 1993

Norden MJ: Fluoxetine in borderline personality disorder. Prog Neuropsychopharmacol Biol Psychiatry 13:218–220, 1989

Nurnberg HG, Raskin M, Levine PE, et al: The comorbidity of borderline personality disorder and other DSM-III-R Axis II personality disorders. Am J Psychiatry 148:1371–1377, 1991

Ogata SN, Silk KR, Goodrich S: The childhood experience of the borderline patient, in Family Environment and Borderline Personality Disorder. Edited by Links PS. Washington, DC, American Psychiatric Press, 1990a, pp 85–103

Ogata SN, Silk KR, Goodrich S, et al: Childhood sexual and physical abuse in adult patients with borderline personality disorder. Am J Psychiatry 147:1008–1013, 1990b

Oldham JM, Skodol AE, Kellman HD, et al: Diagnosis of DSM-III-R personality disorders by two structured interviews: patterns of comorbidity. Am J Psychiatry 149:213–220, 1992

O'Leary KM, Brouwers P, Gardner DL, et al: Neuropsychological testing of patients with borderline personality disorder. Am J Psychiatry 148:106–111, 1991

Paris J: Follow-up studies of borderline personality: a critical review. Journal of Personality Disorders 2:189–197, 1988

Paris J: Personality disorders, parasuicide, and culture. Transcultural Psychiatric Research Review 28:25–40, 1991

Paris J: Social risk factors for borderline personality disorder: a review and hypothesis. Can J Psychiatry 37:510–515, 1992

Paris J: Personality disorders: a biopsychosocial model. Journal of Personality Disorders 7:255–264, 1993a

Paris J: The treatment of borderline personality disorder in light of the research on its long term outcome. Can J Psychiatry 38 (suppl 1):S28–S34, 1993b

Paris J, Frank H: Perceptions of parental bonding in borderline patients. Am J Psychiatry 146:1498–1499, 1989

Paris J, Zweig-Frank H: A critical review of the role of childhood sexual abuse in the etiology of borderline personality disorder. Can J Psychiatry 37:125–128, 1992

Paris J, Zweig-Frank H: Parental bonding in borderline personality disorder, in Borderline Personality Disorder: Etiology and Treatment. Edited by Paris J. Washington, DC, American Psychiatric Press, 1993, pp 141–159

Paris J, Brown R, Nowlis D: Long-term follow-up of borderline patients in a general hospital. Compr Psychiatry 28:530–535, 1987

Paris J, Nowlis D, Brown R: Developmental factors in the outcome of borderline personality disorder. Compr Psychiatry 29:147–150, 1988

Paris J, Nowlis D, Brown R: Predictors of suicide in borderline personality disorder. Can J Psychiatry 34:8–9, 1989

Paris J, Frank H, Buonvino M, et al: Recollections of parental behavior and Axis II cluster diagnosis. Journal of Personality Disorders 5:102–106, 1991

Paris J, Zweig-Frank H, Guzder H: The role of psychological risk factors in recovery from borderline personality disorder. Compr Psychiatry 34:410–413, 1993

Paris J, Zweig-Frank H, Guzder H: Psychological risk factors for borderline personality disorder in female patients. Compr Psychiatry 1994a

Paris J, Zweig-Frank H, Guzder H: Risk factors for borderline personality in male outpatients. J Nerv Ment Dis 182:375–380, 1994b

Parker G: Parental reports of depressives: an investigation of several explanations. J Affect Disord 3:131–140, 1981

Parker GB: Parental Overprotection: A Risk Factor in Psychosocial Development. New York, Grune & Stratton, 1983

Parker GB, Barrett EA, Hickie IB: From nurture to network: examining links between perceptions of parenting received in childhood and social bonds in adulthood. Am J Psychiatry 149:877–885, 1992

Perry JC: Depression in borderline personality disorder: lifetime prevalence at interview and longitudinal course of symptoms. Am J Psychiatry 142:15–21, 1985

Perry JC: Toward the evolution of designer treatments: childhood trauma informs the treatment of borderline personality disorder. Paper presented to the Second International Congress on the Disorders of the Personality, Oslo, Norway, July 1991

Perry JC: Problems and considerations in the valid assessment of personality disorders. Am J Psychiatry 149:1645–1653, 1992

Perry JC, Cooper SH: Psychodynamics, symptoms, and outcome in borderline and antisocial personality disorders and bipolar type II affective disorder, in The Borderline: Current Empirical Research. Edited by McGlashan TH. Washington, DC, American Psychiatric Press, 1985, pp 19–41

Perry S: Treatment time and the borderline patient: an underappreciated strategy. Journal of Personality Disorders 3:230–239, 1989

Peters DS: Child sexual abuse and later psychological problems, in Lasting Effects of Child Sexual Abuse. Edited by Wyatt GE, Powell GJ. Beverly Hills, CA, Sage, 1988, pp 101–117

Pfohl B, Coryell W, Zimmerman M, et al: DSM-III personality disorders: diagnostic overlap and internal consistency of individual DSM-III criteria. Compr Psychiatry 27:21–34, 1986

Plakun EM, Burkhardt PE, Muller JP: 14-year follow-up of borderline and schizotypal personality disorders. Compr Psychiatry 26:448–455, 1985

Plakun EM, Burkhardt PE, Muller JP: Prediction of outcome in borderline personality disorder. Journal of Personality Disorders 5:93–101, 1991

Plomin R, DeFries JC, McClearn GE: Behavioral Genetics: A Primer. New York, WH Freeman, 1990

Pokorny AD: Prediction of suicide in psychiatric patients: report of a prospective study. Arch Gen Psychiatry 40:249–257, 1983

Pollock VE, Briere J, Schneider L, et al: Childhood antecedents of antisocial behavior: parental alcoholism and physical abusiveness. Am J Psychiatry 147:1290–1293, 1990

Pope HG Jr, Jonas JM, Hudson JI, et al: The validity of DSM-III borderline personality disorder: a phenomenologic, family history, treatment response, and long-term follow-up study. Arch Gen Psychiatry 40:23–30, 1983

Reich J, Yates W, Nduaguba M: Prevalence of DSM-III personality disorders in the community. Soc Psychiatry Psychiatr Epidemiol 24:12–16, 1989

Reid WH (ed): The Psychopath: A Comprehensive Study of Antisocial Disorders and Behaviors. New York, Brunner/Mazel, 1978

Rich CL, Runeson BS: Similarities in diagnostic comorbidity between suicide among young people in Sweden and the United States. Acta Psychiatr Scand 86:335–339, 1992

Rich CL, Fowler RC, Fogarty LA, et al: San Diego Suicide Study, III: relationships between diagnoses and stressors. Arch Gen Psychiatry 45:589–592, 1988

Robins E, Guze SB: Establishment of diagnostic validity in psychiatric illness: its application to schizophrenia. Am J Psychiatry 126:983–987, 1970

Robins LN: Deviant Children Grown Up. Baltimore, MD, Williams & Wilkins, 1966

Robins LN, Regier DA (eds): Psychiatric Disorders in America: The Epidemiologic Catchment Area Study. New York, Free Press, 1991

Robins LN, Schoenberg SP, Holmes SJ, et al: Early home environment and retrospective recall: a test for concordance between siblings with and without psychiatric disorders. Am J Orthopsychiatry 55:27–41, 1985

Rockland LH: Supportive Therapy for Borderline Patients: A Dynamic Approach. New York, Guilford, 1992

Ross CA: Epidemiology of multiple personality disorder and dissociation. Psychiatr Clin North Am 14:503–517, 1991

Rowe DC: Environmental and genetic influences on dimensions of perceived parenting: a twin study. Developmental Psychology 17:203–208, 1981

Runeson B, Beskow J: Borderline personality disorder in young Swedish suicides. J Nerv Ment Dis 179:153–156, 1991

Russell DEH: The Secret Trauma: Incest in the Lives of Girls and Women. New York, Basic Books, 1986

Rutter M: Psychosocial resilience and protective mechanisms. Am J Orthopsychiatry 57:316–331, 1987

Rutter M: Pathways from childhood to adult life. J Child Psychol Psychiatry 30:23–51, 1989

Rutter M: Temperament, personality and personality disorder. Br J Psychiatry 150:443–458, 1987

Rutter M, Rutter M: Developing Minds: Challenge and Continuity Across the Life Span. New York, Basic Books, 1993

Sadavoy J: The aging borderline, in The Handbook of Borderline Disorders. Edited by Silver D, Rosenbluth M. New York, International Universities Press, 1992, pp 553–579

Sauzier M: Disclosure of child sexual abuse: for better or for worse. Psychiatr Clin North Am 12:455–469, 1989

Scarr S, McCartney K: How people make their own environments: a theory of genotype-environment effects. Child Dev 54:424–435, 1983

Scarr S, Yee D: Heritability and educational policy: genetic and environmental effects on IQ, aptitude, and achievement. Educational Psychology 15:1–22, 1980

Schmideberg M: The borderline patient, in American Handbook of Psychiatry, Vol 1. Edited by Arieti S. New York, Basic Books, 1959, pp 398–416

Schulz PM, Schulz SC, Goldberg SC, et al: Diagnoses of the relatives of schizotypal outpatients. J Nerv Ment Dis 174:457–463, 1986

Serban G, Siegel S: Response of borderline and schizotypal patients to small doses of thiothixene and haloperidol. Am J Psychiatry 141:1455–1458, 1984

Shea MT, Pilkonis PA, Beckham E, et al: Personality disorders and treatment outcome in the NIMH Treatment of Depression Collaborative Research Program. Am J Psychiatry 147:711–718, 1990

Shearer SL, Peters CP, Quaytman MS, et al: Frequency and correlates of childhood sexual and physical abuse histories in adult female borderline inpatients. Am J Psychiatry 147:214–216, 1990

Shearin EN, Linehan MM: Dialectical behavior therapy for borderline personality disorder: treatment goals, strategies, and empirical support, in Borderline Personality Disorder: Etiology and Treatment. Edited by Paris J. Washington, DC, American Psychiatric Press, 1993, pp 285–318

Siever LJ: A psychobiological model of personality disorders. Paper presented to the International Society for the Study of Personality Disorders, Cambridge, MA, September 1993

Siever LJ, Davis KL: A psychobiological perspective on the personality disorders. Am J Psychiatry 148:1647–1658, 1991

Sigal JJ, Weinfeld M: Trauma and Rebirth: Intergenerational Effects of the Holocaust. New York, Praeger, 1989

Silk KR, Eisner W, Demars C, et al: Interrupted inpatient treatment of borderlines. Paper presented at the 145th annual meeting of the American Psychiatric Association, Washington, DC, May 1992

Silk KR, Karle B, Lohr N, et al: Sexual abuse and family environment in BPD. Paper presented at the 146th annual meeting of the American Psychiatric Association, San Francisco, CA, May 1993

Silver D: Psychotherapy of the characterologically difficult patient. Can J Psychiatry 28:513–521, 1983

Silver D: Psychodynamics and psychotherapeutic management of the self-destructive character-disordered patient. Psychiatr Clin North Am 8:357–375, 1985

Silver D, Cardish RJ: BPD outcome studies: psychotherapy implications. Paper presented at the 144th annual meeting of the American Psychiatric Association, New Orleans, LA, May 1991

Silver D, Rosenbluth MA: Inpatient treatment of borderline personality disorder, in Borderline Personality Disorder: Etiology and Treatment. Edited by Paris J. Washington, DC, American Psychiatric Press, 1993, pp 349–372

Silverman JM, Pinkham L, Horvath TB, et al: Affective and impulsive personality disorder traits in the relatives of patients with borderline personality disorder. Am J Psychiatry 148:1378–1385, 1991

Simonsen E: Prevalence of BPD in Europe. Paper presented at the 146th annual meeting of the American Psychiatric Association, San Francisco, CA, May 1993

Skodol AE, Buckley P, Charles E: Is there a characteristic pattern to the treatment history of clinic outpatients with borderline personality? J Nerv Ment Dis 171:405–410, 1983

Smith ML, Glass GV, Miller TI: The Benefits of Psychotherapy. Baltimore, MD, Johns Hopkins University Press, 1980

Soldz S, Budman S, Dembry A, et al: Representation of personality disorders in circumplex and five-factor space: exploration with a clinical sample. Psychological Assessment 5:41–52, 1993

Soloff PH: What's new in personality disorders? An update on pharmacological treatment. Journal of Personality Disorders 4:233–243, 1990

Soloff PH: Pharmacological therapies in borderline personality disorder, in Borderline Personality Disorder: Etiology and Treatment. Edited by Paris J. Washington, DC, American Psychiatric Press, 1993, pp 319–348

Soloff PH, Millward JW: Developmental histories of borderline patients. Compr Psychiatry 24:574–588, 1983a

Soloff PH, Millward JW: Psychiatric disorders in the families of borderline patients. Arch Gen Psychiatry 40:37–44, 1983b

Soloff PH, George A, Nathan RS, et al: Paradoxical effects of amitriptyline on borderline patients. Am J Psychiatry 143:1603–1605, 1986

Southwick SM, Yehuda R, Giller EL Jr, et al: Altered platelet α_2-adrenergic receptor binding sites in borderline personality disorder. Am J Psychiatry 147:1014–1017, 1990

Spitzer RL, Endicott J, Gibbon M: Crossing the border into borderline personality and borderline schizophrenia. Arch Gen Psychiatry 36:17–24, 1979

Stein G: Drug treatment of the personality disorders. Br J Psychiatry 161:167–184, 1992

Stelmack RM: Advances in personality theory and research. Journal of Psychiatry and Neuroscience 16:131–138, 1991

Stern A: Psychoanalytic investigation of and therapy in the border line group of neuroses. Psychoanal Q 7:467–489, 1938

Stevenson J, Meares R: An outcome study of psychotherapy for patients with borderline personality disorder. Am J Psychiatry 149:358–362, 1992

Stone MH: The Borderline Syndromes: Constitution, Personality, and Adaptation. New York, McGraw-Hill, 1980

Stone MH: Psychotherapy of borderline patients in light of long-term follow-up. Bull Menninger Clin 51:231–247, 1987

Stone MH: The Fate of Borderline Patients: Successful Outcome and Psychiatric Practice. New York, Guilford, 1990

Stone MH: Etiology of borderline personality disorder: psychobiological factors contributing to an underlying irritability, in Borderline Personality Disorder: Etiology and Treatment. Edited by Paris J. Washington, DC, American Psychiatric Press, 1993a, pp 87–101

Stone MH: Long-term outcome in personality disorders. Br J Psychiatry 162:299–313, 1993b

Strupp HH, Hadley SW: Specific vs nonspecific factors in psychotherapy: a controlled study of outcome. Arch Gen Psychiatry 36:1125–1136, 1979

Strupp HH, Fox RE, Lessler K: Patients View Their Psychotherapy. Baltimore, MD, Johns Hopkins Press, 1969

Sudak HS, Ford AB, Rushforth NB (eds): Suicide in the Young. Boston, MA, John Wright, 1984

Svrakic DM, Whitehead C, Przybeck TR, et al: Differential diagnosis of personality disorders by the seven-factor model of temperament and character. Arch Gen Psychiatry 50:991–999, 1993

Swartz M, Blazer D, George L, et al: Estimating the prevalence of borderline personality disorder in the community. Journal of Personality Disorders 4:257–272, 1990

Swett C Jr, Surrey J, Cohen C: Sexual and physical abuse histories and psychiatric symptoms among male psychiatric outpatients. Am J Psychiatry 147:632–636, 1990

Taylor C: The Malaise of Modernity. Toronto, Anisna, 1992

Teicher MH, Glod CA, Aaronson ST, et al: Open assessment of the safety and efficacy of thioridazine in the treatment of patients with borderline personality disorder. Psychopharmacol Bull 25:535–549, 1989

Teicher MH, Glod C[A], Cole JO: Emergence of intense suicidal preoccupation during fluoxetine treatment. Am J Psychiatry 147:207–210, 1990

Tellegen A, Lykken DT, Bouchard TJ, et al: Personality similarity in twins reared apart and together. J Pers Soc Psychol 54:1031–1039, 1988

Tennant C: Parental loss in childhood: its effect in adult life. Arch Gen Psychiatry 45:1045–1050, 1988

Thompson RA, Connell JP, Bridges LJ: Temperament, emotion, and social interactive behavior in the strange situation. Child Dev 56:1106–1110, 1988

Thorslund J: Inuit suicide in Greenland. Arctic Med Res 49:25–33, 1990

Torgersen S: The oral, obsessive, and hysterical personality syndromes: a study of hereditary and environmental factors by means of the twin method. Arch Gen Psychiatry 37:1272–1277, 1980

Torgersen S: Genetic factors in anxiety disorders. Arch Gen Psychiatry 40:1085–1089, 1983

Torgersen S: Genetic and nosological aspects of schizotypal and borderline personality disorders: a twin study. Arch Gen Psychiatry 41:546–554, 1984

Torgersen S: Heritability of the DSM personality disorders. Paper presented to the International Society for the Study of Personality Disorders, Cambridge, MA, September 1993

Torgersen S, Alnæs R: Localizing DSM-III personality disorders in a three-dimensional structural space. Journal of Personality Disorders 3:274–281, 1989

Torgersen S, Alnæs R: Differential perception of parental bonding in schizotypal and borderline personality disorders. Compr Psychiatry 33:34–38, 1992

Torgersen S, Skre I, Onstad J, et al: The psychometric-genetic structure of DSM-III-R personality disorder diagnostic criteria. Journal of Personality Disorders 7:196–213, 1993

Tyrer P: Personality Disorders: Diagnosis, Management, and Course. Boston, MA, John Wright, 1988

Tyrer P: Categorical and dimensional approaches to personality disorders. Paper presented to the Association for Research on Personality Disorders, San Francisco, CA, May 1993

Vaillant GE: A 20-year follow-up of New York narcotic addicts. Arch Gen Psychiatry 29:237–241, 1973

Vaillant GE: Adaptation to Life. Boston, MA, Little, Brown, 1977

Vaillant GE: The Natural History of Alcoholism. Cambridge, MA, Harvard University Press, 1983

van der Kolk BA, Perry JC, Herman JL: Childhood origins of self-destructive behavior. Am J Psychiatry 148:1665–1671, 1991

van Reekum R, Links PS, Boiago I: Constitutional factors in borderline personality disorder: genetics, brain dysfunction, and biological markers, in Borderline Personality Disorder: Etiology and Treatment. Edited by Paris J. Washington, DC, American Psychiatric Press, 1993, pp 13–38

Wachtel P: Psychoanalysis and Behavior Therapy: Toward an Integration. New York, Basic Books, 1977

Waldinger RJ: Intensive psychodynamic therapy with borderline patients: an overview. Am J Psychiatry 144:267–274, 1987

Waldinger RJ, Frank AF: Clinicians' experiences in combining medication and psychotherapy in the treatment of borderline patients. Hosp Community Psychiatry 40:712–718, 1989

Waldinger RJ, Gunderson JG: Completed psychotherapies with borderline patients. Am J Psychother 38:190–202, 1984

Waldinger RJ, Gunderson JG: Effective Psychotherapy With Borderline Patients: Case Studies. New York, Macmillan, 1987

Wallerstein J: Second Chances: Men, Women, and Children a Decade After Divorce. New York, Ticknor & Fields, 1989

Weiner H: Psychobiology and Human Disease. New York, Elsevier, 1977

Weissman MM: The epidemiology of suicide attempts, 1960 to 1971. Arch Gen Psychiatry 30:737–746, 1974

Werble B: Second follow-up study of borderline patients. Arch Gen Psychiatry 23:3–7, 1970

Westen D: Self and Society: Narcissism, Collectivism and the Development of Morals. New York, Cambridge University Press, 1985

Westen D, Ludolph P, Misle B, et al: Physical and sexual abuse in adolescent girls with borderline personality disorder. Am J Orthopsychiatry 60:55–66, 1990

Wiggins JS: Circumplex models of interpersonal behavior in clinical psychology, in Handbook of Research Methods in Clinical Psychology. Edited by Kendall PS, Butcher JN. New York, Wiley, 1982, pp 183–221

Wiggins JS, Pincus AL: Conceptions of personality disorders and dimensions of personality. Psychological Assessment 1:305–316, 1989

Wilkinson DG: The suicide rate in schizophrenia. Br J Psychiatry 140:138–141, 1982

Wilson EO: Sociobiology. Cambridge, MA, Belknap Press/Harvard University Press, 1975

Winnicott DW: Collected Papers. New York, International Universities Press, 1964

Wolberg AR: The Borderline Patient. New York, Intercontinental Medical, 1973

World Health Organization: International Classification of Diseases, 10th Revision. Geneva, World Health Organization, 1992

Wyatt G: The sexual abuse of Afro-American and white women in childhood. Child Abuse Negl 9:507–519, 1985

Yalom ID: The Theory and Practice of Group Psychotherapy, 3rd Edition. New York, Basic Books, 1985

Yochelson S, Samenow SE: The Criminal Personality. New York, Jason Aronson, 1976

Zanarini MC: Borderline personality disorder as an impulse spectrum disorder, in Borderline Personality Disorder: Etiology and Treatment. Edited by Paris J. Washington, DC, American Psychiatric Press, 1993a, pp 67–85

Zanarini MC: Two- to six-year follow-ups of borderline outpatients and Axis II controls. Paper presented to the International Society for the Study of Personality Disorders, Cambridge, MA, September 1993b

Zanarini MC, Gunderson JG, Frankenburg FR: The Revised Diagnostic Interview for Borderlines: discriminating BPD from other Axis II disorders. Journal of Personality Disorders 3:10–18, 1989a

Zanarini MC, Gunderson JG, Marino MF, et al: Childhood experiences of borderline patients. Compr Psychiatry 30:18–25, 1989b

Zanarini MC, Gunderson JG, Frankenburg FR: Cognitive features of borderline personality disorder. Am J Psychiatry 147:57–63, 1990a

Zanarini MC, Gunderson JG, Frankenburg FR, et al: Discriminating borderline personality disorder from other Axis II disorders. Am J Psychiatry 147:161–167, 1990b

Zanarini MC, Dubo ED, Lewis RE, et al: The relationship between sexual abuse and BPD. Paper presented at the 146th annual meeting of the American Psychiatric Association, San Francisco, CA, May 1993

Zetzel ER: A developmental approach to the borderline patient. Am J Psychiatry 127:867–871, 1971

Zimmerman M, Jampala VC, Sierles FS, et al: DSM-IV: a nosology sold before its time? Am J Psychiatry 148:463–467, 1991

Zuckerman J: Sensation Seeking: Beyond the Optimum Level of Arousal. Hillsdale, NJ, Lawrence Erlbaum, 1979

Zweig-Frank H, Paris J: Parents' emotional neglect and overprotection according to the recollections of patients with borderline personality disorder. Am J Psychiatry 148:648–651, 1991

Zweig-Frank H, Paris J, Guzder J: Psychological risk factors for dissociation and self-mutilation in female patients with borderline personality disorder. Can J Psychiatry 1994a

Zweig-Frank H, Paris J, Guzder J: Psychological risk factors for self-mutilation in male patients with borderline personality disorder. Can J Psychiatry 1994b

Zweig-Frank H, Paris J, Guzder J: Dissociation in borderline and non-borderline personality disorders. Journal of Personality Disorders (in press)

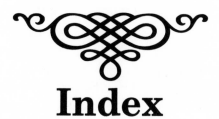

Index

*Page numbers printed in **boldface** type refer to tables or figures.*

Abnormal parenting
  affectionless control and, 65
  biparental failure and, 65
  as BPD outcome predictor, 102
  extrafamilial relationships and,
    77
  "goodness of fit" concept and,
    89, 92
  multivariate risk factors with,
    66–68
  parental bonding and, 62–66
  Parental Bonding Index (PBI)
    and, 44–45, 64–65
  parental psychopathology and,
    61–62
  physical, verbal abuse and
    family violence, 58–60
  social factors affecting, 76–77,
    96–97
Active-passive polarity, 15
Adaptive personality traits, 32–35
Affectionless control by parents,
  65

Affective instability
  biological risk factors and,
    40–41
  BPD comorbid diagnosis with,
    8
  BPD core dimension of, xvi,
    21–22, 23–25, 94–95, 156
  BPD outcome predictor of, 102
  in BPD parents, 61–62
  BPD symptom of, 2
  maturation and, xvii, 105
  mood disorders confused with, 5
  social disintegration and, 83
  treatment of
    carbamazepine used,
      114–115
    mechanisms for, 128–130
    pharmacological, 110
    tranylcypromine used, 113
Agreeableness
  BPD patient scores on, 21
  Costa and McCrae personality
    theory and, 15

Alcoholism
  of BPD parents, 61
  cross-cultural comparisons of,
    70–71
  maturation and, 105
  prevalence, increase of, 74
Alliance formation in
    psychotherapy, 135–136
  case studies of, 143–146
Amitriptyline treatment, 113
Antidepressant treatment, 113
Antisocial personality disorder
    (ASPD)
  appropriate adaptive situations
    for, 33
  BPD overlap with, 74
  childhood physical abuse and, 59
  gender differences in, 24
  maturation and, 104
  parental psychopathology and,
    61, 66
  prevalence and social class
    distribution of, 72
  social risk factors in, 70
ASPD. *See* Antisocial personality
    disorder (ASPD)
Attachment theory of parental
    bonding, 62–63, 90
Axis I disorders
  biological vulnerability and, 28
  BPD delimited from, 6–7
  comorbid diagnosis from, 7–8
  single required criterion and, 5
Axis II disorders
  biological vulnerability and,
    28–29

BPD delimited from, 6–7
diagnosis through interviews
    of, 4
dimensional personality theory
    diagnosis of, 18–19

Benzodiazepine treatment, 115
Biological personality theory
  Cloninger model, 15–16
  Millon model, 15
Biological risk factors, 25
  See also Biopsychosocial
    theory; Neurotransmitter
    systems; Twin studies
  adaptive, maladaptive
    personality traits and,
    32–35
  BPD core dimensions and,
    31–32, 40–41
  genetics of personality and,
    29–31
  paradigms and personality
    disorders, 27–29
  research on, 156–157
  vulnerability, evidence of,
    35–38
Biological vulnerability
  See also Biological risk factors
  as basis of neo-Kraepelinian
    paradigm, xiv–xv
  depression and, 8–9
  evidence of, 35–38
  heritability of, xvi
  neurophysiological
    disturbances and, 37–38
  personality traits and, 11, 24–25

Biopsychosocial theory
  of BPD, 93–97, **94**
    core dimensions of, 93–95
    multidimensional,
      interactive model of,
      96–97
    of personality traits, disorders, **88**
    biological factors and, 89
    environmental unshared
      variance and, 89–90
    psychological factors and, 90
    social learning theory and,
      90–91
    temperament and, 88–89
  research on, 158–159
Biparental failure, 65
Borderline personality disorder
  (BPD)
  See also Affective instability;
    Biological vulnerability;
    Biopsychosocial theory;
    Clinical management;
    Impulsivity, impulsive
    disorders; Psychological
    risk factors; Social risk
    factors; Treatment options
  biopsychosocial approach to,
    xiii–xiv, **94**
  comorbidity and, 7–9
  core dimensions of, xvi, 20–23
    affective instability, xvi, 22,
      23–25, 94–95, 156
    cognitive impairment, 22, 23
    identity diffusion, 22
    impulsivity, xvi, 22, 23–25,
      94–95, 156

definition of terms, 1–2
diagnosis, operational criteria
  for, 2–5
diagnostic interview for, 4
gender differences in, 24, 46
increasing prevalence of, 73–74
multidimensional approach to,
  xii–xiii, xvii
outcome of
  change mechanisms and,
    104–105
  clinical management
    implications and,
    105–107
  global outcome and suicide,
    99–104
  recovery from, 101
  risk factors and, 25
  social disintegration and,
    82–83
symptoms of, 1–2
syndrome vs. disorder
  terminology, 6–7
validity of, 5–7
Borderline personality
  organization (BPO), 20
BPD. *See* Borderline personality
  disorder (BPD)
BPO. *See* Borderline personality
  organization (BPO)
Buss and Plomin dimensional
  personality theory, **14**, 15

Carbamazepine treatment,
  114–115, 142
Catecholamine activity, 38–39

Categorical approach to
   personality disorders, 19–20
CBT. *See* Cognitive-behavior
   therapy (CBT)
Childhood dimensional
   personality model
   Buss and Plomin, 15
   dissociation and, 56–57
   self mutilation and, 57–58
Childhood sexual abuse
   BPD and, 51–55
      linkage mechanisms of,
         55–56
      as outcome predictor, 102
      symptoms as abuse markers,
         56–58
   defense mechanisms and, 58
   family dysfunction and, 56, 62
   feminist-inspired research and,
      45–46
   gender differences and, 46, 54
   incest vs. molestation, 48–49
   multivariate risk factors with,
      66–68
   parameters of, 46–47
      age at onset, 49
      disclosure and, 49
      frequency, duration and,
         47–48
      relationship to the
         perpetrator, 48–49
      severity of, 48
      statistics of, 49–51
Cholinergic system, 38
Circumplex interpersonal
   personality theory, 17

Clinical management
   of BPD, 105–107
   guidelines for, 133–134
   treatment and
      competence as aim of,
         148–151
      intermittent treatment,
         151–153
      role of structure in, 146–148
      symptom control, 139–146
      treatability determination,
         134–139
Cloninger biological dimensional
   personality theory, **14**, 15–16,
   35
Cognitive impairment
   biological risk factors and, 40
   BPD dimension of, 22, 23
Cognitive processing of childhood
   sexual abuse, 55
Cognitive-behavior therapy
   (CBT)
   dialectical behavior therapy
      (DBT) and, 122–124, 140
   parental failure and, 63
Comorbidity explanation vs.
   artifact, 7–9
Competence-oriented treatment
   approach, 148–151
Conscientiousness
   BPD patients' scores on, 21
   Costa and McCrae personality
      theory and, 15
   impulsivity facet of, 22
   Tellegen personality theory
      and, 17

Constraint, Tellegen personality
theory and, 17
Costa and McCrae dimensional
personality theory, **14**, 15
personality disorder measured
by, 18
Cultural factors
alcoholism and, 70–71
eating disorders and, 71
impulsivity affected by, 74–75
social risk factors and, 70,
74–75
suicide and, 75
youth suicide and, 75, 79

Day treatment, 115–117
DBT. *See* Dialectical behavior
therapy (DBT)
Defense mechanisms of childhood
sexual abuse, 58
Defense Style Questionnaire, 58
Depression
biological and environmental
triggers of, 2–9
BPD comorbid diagnosis from, 8
in BPD parents, 61, 62
childhood sexual abuse and, 47
multiple risk factors in, xiii
parental dysfunction and, 64
pharmacological treatment of,
114
social risk factors in, 70
DES. *See* Dissociative Experiences
Scale (DES)
Diagnosis, operational criteria,
2–5

Diagnostic Index for Borderlines
(DIB), 100, 101
Diagnostic Interview for
Borderlines, 4, 52
*Diagnostic and Statistical Manual of
Mental Disorders. See* DSM;
DSM-I; DSM-II; DSM-III;
DSM-IV
Dialectical behavior therapy
(DBT), 122–124, 140
group therapy and, 127
DIB. *See* Diagnostic Index for
Borderlines (DIB)
Dimensional theories of
personality
models of, **14**, 20–23
Buss and Plomin model, **14**,
15
Clarkin and Kernberg
model, 20
Cloninger model, **14**, 15–16
Costa and McCrae model,
14, 15
Eysenck model, **14**, 13–15
Leary and Wiggins model,
14, 17
Livesley model, 17, 20
Millon model, **14**, 15
Siever and Davis model, **14**,
22, 23–24
multidimensional schemas of, 17
personality disorder diagnosis
by, 18–19
Tellegen model, **14**, 17
Dissociation of childhood sexual
abuse, 56–57

Dissociative Experiences Scale (DES), 57
Dizygotic twins. *See* Twin studies
Dopaminergic activity
  cognitive impairment and, 40
  extroversion and, 14, 16
DSM-III
  BPD in, xv, 3, 4
  personality disorders, 19
  posttraumatic stress disorder (PTSD) in, 45
DSM-IV
  BPD in, 4
  clinical trials vs. research findings, 5–7
  criteria, basis of, 5–7
  personality disorders, 19

Eating disorders in cross-cultural comparisons, 71
Ego strength
  case study of
    negative alliance formation, 138, 142
    positive alliance formation, 137–138
  as psychotherapy alliance indicator, 136
Environment of evolutionary adaptiveness, 33
  temperament, traits, disorders and, 87–93
Environmental risk factors
  See also Biopsychosocial theory
  biological vulnerability combined with, 29, 31

depression and, 8–9
trait-linked behaviors and, 95
twin studies and, 30–31
unshared variance and, 89–90
Epidemiologic Catchment Area (ECA) study
  of antisocial personality disorder, 71
  of childhood sexual abuse, 50
Extroversion
  BPD patients scores on, 21
  Buss and Plomin personality theory and, 15
  Cloninger personality theory and, 16
  Costa and McCrae personality theory and, 15
  environmental risk factors and, 92–93
  Eysenck personality theory and, 13, 89
  Tellegen personality theory and, 17
Eysenck Personality Inventory (EPI), 21, 89
Eyseneck personality theory, 13–15, **14**, 89

Family dysfunction
  of BPD patients, 62
  childhood sexual abuse and, 56, 62
Family Environment Scale measurement of, 62
  separation and loss and, 61
Family Environment Scale, 62

Family structure
  extrafamilial relationships and,
    77
  of immigrant families, 84
  social factors affecting, 96–97
    rapid social change, 76–77,
      80–81, 84
    social disintegration, 81–82
    social learning theory and,
      90–91
Family studies
  See also Heritability
  of affective disorders, 35–36
  of impulsive disorders, 7, 24,
    35–36
  of mood disorders, 8
  of substance abuse, 35
Family violence, as psychological
  risk factor, 58–60
Fenfluramine challenge test, 36
Fertility. *See* Reproduction
Fluoxetine treatment, 114

GAS. *See* Global Assessment
  Scale (GAS)
Gender differences
  in BPD, 24, 46
  in childhood physical abuse,
    59–60
  in parental dysfunction, 65–66
Global Assessment Scale (GAS),
  100, 101
"Goodness of fit" parenting
  concept, 89, 92
Greenland, rapid acculturation, 79
Group therapy, 127

Harm avoidance
  BPD patient scores on, 21
  Cloninger personality theory
    and, 16
Health-Sickness Rating Scale
  (HSRS), 100, 101
Heritability
  See also Biological risk factors;
    Biological vulnerability;
    Family studies; Twin studies
  of biological vulnerability, xvi
  dimensional personality theory
    testing of, 16
  of intelligence, 29
  twin studies and, 30–31, 36
Hospitalization treatment,
  115–117
HSRS. *See* Health-Sickness
  Rating Scale (HSRS)
Hypersensitivity, 2

Identity formation
  BPD dimension of, 21, 22, 23
  social risk factors affecting, 80,
    83
Imaginativeness, 15
Immigrant family structure, 84
Impulsivity, impulsive disorders
  See also specific behavior
  adaptive/maladaptive
    continuum of, 33
  biological risk factors and,
    40–41
  BPD core dimension of, xvi,
    21–22, 23–25, 94–95, 156
  of BPD parents, 61

Impulsivity, impulsive disorders
(*continued*)
cultural factors affecting, 74–75
Eysenck personality theory
and, 13
female sexual impulsivity and,
33–34
gender differences in, 24
maturation and, xvii, 104–105,
144–146
as neuroticism,
conscientiousness facet, 22
parental dysfunction and, 63–64
prevalence, increase of, 73–74
research on, 71–72
serotonin activity and, 16, 23,
36–37, 39
social disintegration and,
78–79, 81–83
symptom control of, 140–146
symptom of, 2, 5
treatment of, 109–110, 120
carbamazepine used, 115
dialectical behavior therapy
(DBT) and, 123–124
hospitalization, 116
mechanisms of, 128–130
neuroleptics used, 112–113,
140
supportive psychotherapy
and, 125
Incest
family dysfunction and, 56
perpetrator relationship and,
48–49
statistics on, 49–51, 52

Inferiority, 2
Intelligence
BPD outcome related to, 102
classification of, 19
heritability of, 29
International Classification of
Diseases, 3–4
Interpersonal personality theory
Benjamin model of, 17
Lear and Wiggins model of, 17
Interpersonal relationships. *See*
Relationships, instability of
Introjection of psychotherapy, 118

Lability dimension of BPD, 21,
23–24
Leary and Wiggins dimensional
personality theory, **14**, 17
Limbic system, 14
Lithium treatment, 114

Maladaptive personality traits,
32–35
Masochism, 2
Maturation, disorders affected by,
xvii, 104–105, 144–146
Millon dimensional personality
theory, **14**, 15
Monoamine oxidase inhibitor
treatment, 113
Monozygotic twins. *See* Twin
studies
Multidimensional approach,
xii–xiii, xvii
Multidimensional theory. *See*
Biopsychosocial theory

Narcissism, 1
Native American, rapid
    acculturation, 79
Neo-Kraepelinian paradigm
    biological vulnerability and,
        xiv–xv, 28–29
    "borderline" terminology and, 3
    comorbidity and, 7
NEO-PI, 15, 18
    BPD patients measured by, 21
Neuroleptic impulsivity
    treatment, 112–113, 140
Neurophysiological disturbances.
    See also Neurotransmitter
    systems
    measurement of, 37–38
Neuroticism
    Buss and Plomin personality
        theory and, 15
    Costa and McCrae personality
        theory and, 15
    Eysenck personality theory
        and, 13, 14–15
    impulsivity facet of, 22
    maturation and, 104
    measured in BPD patients, 21
Neurotransmitter systems
    behavior, relationship to, 16
    biological treatment of, 108
    maturation and, 105
    noradrenergic system and, 23
    norepinephrine and, 38–39
    personality disorders and, 28,
        38–39
    serotonin activity and, 16, 23,
        36–37, 39

Noradrenergic system, 23
Norepinephrine
    affective instability and, 38,
        39
    reward dependence and, 16

Overprotection of children,
    63–64, 65

Paranoia case study, 135
Parasuicide. *See* Suicide, suicide
    attempts
Parental Bonding Index (PBI),
    44–45, 64–65
Parents. *See* Abnormal parenting
PBI. *See* Parental bonding Index
    (PBI)
Personality dimensions
    See also Dimensional theories
        of personality
    of BPD, 20–23
    vs. categories in classification,
        19–20
    personality theories and, 14–17
    personality trait intensity and,
        12
    research on, 156
    social risk factors and, 76
Personality disorders
    biopsychosocial theory of,
        88–93, **88**
    categorical vs. dimensional
        approach to, 19–20
    dimensional diagnostic
        methods of, 18–19
    risk factors in, 25

Personality disorders *(continued)*
  social risk factors in
    prevalence, social class
      distribution of, 72–73
    research strategies of, 71–72
  traits vs. temperament and, 11,
    88–89
Personality theories. *See*
  Dimensional theories of
  personality
Personality traits
  See also Biological risk factors;
    Biological vulnerability;
    Family studies; Twin studies
  adaptive vs. maladaptive,
    32–35
  biological vulnerability and,
    11, 24–25, 28–29, 29–31
  biopsychosocial theory of,
    88–93, **88**
  categories and dimensions of,
    12
  dimensional personality
    theories and, 12–17
  genetics of, 29–31
  intensity measurement of, 11
  research on, 156–157
  risk factors and, 25
  vs. temperament, 11, 88–89
PET. *See* Positron-emission
  tomography (PET)
Pharmacological interventions,
  112–115
  antidepressants used, 113
  neuroleptics used, 112–113
  overdose, risk of, 114

specific serotonin reuptake
    inhibitors (SSRIs) used,
    113–114
Phobias, 33
Physical abuse, as psychological
  risk factor, 58–60
Pleasure-pain polarity, 15
Positron-emission tomography
  (PET), 37
Posttraumatic stress disorder
  (PTSD)
  BPD theory and, 9, 46
  dissociation and, 56
  feminist-inspired research and,
    45–46
  war veteran experiences and,
    45
Projection, 2
Prospective vs. retrospective
  studies, 44–45, 47
  on BPD suicide tendencies,
    103–104
Psychodynamic theory
  See also Treatment options,
    psychotherapy
  personality traits shaping and,
    90
  psychotherapy for BPD, xviii,
    117–122
Psychoeducation, in treatment of
  impulsivity, 140
Psychological risk factors, 25
  See also Biopsychosocial theory
  abnormal parenting and
    affectionless control and, 65
  biparental failure and, 65

as BPD outcome predictor,
102
extrafamilial relationships
and, 77
"goodness of fit" concept
and, 89, 92
multivariate risk factors
with, 66–68
parental bonding and, 62–66
Parental Bonding Index
(PBI) and, 44–45, 64–65
parental psychopathology
and, 61–62
physical, verbal abuse and
family violence, 58–60
social factors affecting,
76–77, 96–97
biological vulnerability
combined with, 32
childhood sexual abuse
BPD and, 51–55
BPD linkage mechanisms to,
55–56
BPD symptoms as markers
for abuse, 56–58
parameters of, 46–49
statistics of, 49–51
childhood trauma and, xvi,
45–46
measurement methodology
issues of, 43–45
Parental bonding Index
(PBI) and, 44–45, 64–65
multivariate findings on, 66–68
research on, 157–158
separation and loss, 60–61

trait-linked behaviors and,
91–92, 94–95
Psychotherapy, 125–126
See also Treatment options,
psychotherapy
alliance formation in, 135–136
attrition from, 122, 135
classical psychoanalysis and,
119, 121
importance of structure in,
118–120
method effectiveness and, 111
psychodynamic therapy and,
118–122
Psychoticism, 13, 15
PTSD. *See* Posttraumatic stress
disorder (PTSD)

Reality-testing difficulties, 2
Relationship management
therapy (RMT), 127
Relationships, instability of
case studies of, 150–151
childhood sexual abuse and, 47
environmental risk factors and,
8–9
maturation and, 105
as psychotherapy alliance
indicator, 136–137
relationship management
therapy (RMT), 127
social risk factors affecting, 83
symptom of, 2, 5
treatment mechanisms for,
128–129
Reproduction dysfunction, 32, 35

Research directions
  of biological risk factors,
    156–157
  of BPD dimensions, 156
  definition, boundaries of,
    155–156
  of multidimensional studies,
    158–159
  outcome research, 159–160
  of psychological risk factors,
    157–158
  of social risk factors, 158
  strategies of, 71–72
  of treatment, 160–61
Reticular activating system, 14
Retrospective vs. prospective
    studies, 44–45, 47
Revictimization of sexually
    abused children, 54
Reward dependence
  BPD patient scores on, 21
  Cloninger personality theory
    and, 16
RMT. *See* Relationship
    management therapy (RMT)

San Diego Suicide Study, 74
SASB. *See* Structural Analysis of
    Social Behavior (SASB)
Schizophrenia
  attention-cognition
    disturbances and, 39, 40
  multiple risk factors in, xiii
  psychoeducational treatment
    of, 124, 140
  term misuse and, 1

Self-mutilation
  as BPD outcome predictor, 102
  as childhood sexual abuse
    marker, 57–58
Separation and loss, as
    psychological risk factor,
    60–61
  suicide predisposition and,
    103
Serotonin activity
  impulsivity, harm avoidance
    and, 16, 23, 36–37
  specific serotonin reuptake
    inhibitor treatment,
    113–114
Sertraline treatment, 114
Sexual impulsivity, 33–34
Siever and Davis personality
    theory model, **14**, 22, 28, 39,
    40
Sociability
  Buss and Plomin personality
    theory and, 15
  and relation of personality trait
    to disorder, 94–95
Social class. *See* Socioeconomic
    class
Social disintegration
  BPD and, 82–83
  family structure affected by,
    81–82
  rapid social change and, 79–81
  as risk factor for impulsive
    personality disorder, 78–79
Social learning theory of child
    development, 90–91

Social risk factors, 25
See also Biopsychosocial theory;
    Social disintegration
cultural factors and, 70, 74–75
influence, mechanisms of,
    75–76
    on family structure,
        function, 76–77
    on personality dimensions, 76
    on social role development,
        77–78
in mental disorders, 69–71
in personality disorders
    prevalence, social class
        distribution of, 72–73
    research strategies of, 71–72
prevalence, increase of, 73–74
research on, 158
social disintegration and, xvii
tests of, 83–84
Social role development, 77–78
Socioeconomic class
BPD distribution among, 72–73
mental disorder prevalence in,
    70
suicide and, 103
Somatic anxiety, symptom of, 2
Structural Analysis of Social
    Behavior (SASB), 17
Subject-object polarity, 15
Substance abuse
as BPD outcome predictor, 102
childhood physical abuse and,
    59
childhood sexual abuse and, 47
maturation and, 104

prevalence, increase of, 74
social risk factors in, 70, 79
youth suicide and, 74, 103
Suicide, suicide attempts, 22
See also Impulsivity, impulsive
    disorders; Youth suicide
BPD global outcome and,
    101–104
BPD prevalence increase and,
    73–74
case study of
    alliance formation, 143–146
    high ego strength, 137–138
    hospitalization, 141–142
    low ego strength, 138, 142
    structured treatment, 147–148
childhood physical abuse and,
    59
childhood sexual abuse and, 47
cultural factors affecting, 75
day treatment of, 117
dialectical behavior therapy
    (DBT) and, 123–124
gender differences in, 24
hospitalization and, 115–116
social risk factors in, 70, 82
symptom control of, 140–146
Supportive psychotherapy. See
    Psychotherapy

Tellegen dimensional personality
    theory, **14**, 17
Temperament
abnormal attachment and, 90
parental shaping of, 89, 91, 92
vs. personality traits, 11, 88–89

TPQ. *See* Tridimensional
　　Personality Questionnaire
　　(TPQ)
Traits. *See* Personality traits
Transient stress-related reactions,
　　5
Tranylcypromine treatment, 113
Trauma. *See* Abnormal
　　parenting; Childhood
　　sexual abuse; Posttraumatic
　　stress disorder (PTSD);
　　Separation and loss
Traumatic risk factors, xvi
Treatment options, 109–10
　　See also Clinical management
　　clinical trials, caveats and
　　　　population heterogeneity,
　　　　111–112
　　　　sampling problems, 110–111
　　　　specific and nonspecific
　　　　　effects of, 111
　　cognitive-behavior therapy
　　　　(CBT), 122–124
　　day treatment, 115–117, 140
　　　　case study of, 142
　　dialectical behavior therapy
　　　　(DBT), 122–124
　　group therapy, 127
　　hospitalization, xvii, 115–117,
　　　　140–141
　　　　case study of, 141
　　no treatment, 127–128
　　psychopharmacological
　　　　interventions, xvii
　　　　antidepressants used, 113
　　　　benzodiazepines used, 115

　　　　carbamazepine used,
　　　　　114–115, 142
　　　　lithium used, 114
　　　　neuroleptics used, 112–113
　　　　serotonin reuptake
　　　　　inhibitors used, 113–114
　　psychotherapy, xvii–xviii,
　　　　117–122
　　　　attrition from, 122
　　　　case study of
　　　　　alliance formation,
　　　　　　143–146
　　　　　competence formation,
　　　　　　148–151
　　　　　high ego strength, 137–138
　　　　　low ego strength, 138
　　　　classical psychoanalysis and,
　　　　　119, 121
　　　　intermittent, 126, 151–153
　　　　method effectiveness and,
　　　　　111
　　　　psychodynamic therapy and,
　　　　　118–122
　　　　structure importance in,
　　　　　118–120
　　　　supportive, 125–126
　　research on, 160–161
　　successful treatment
　　　　mechanisms, 128–130
Tridimensional Personality
　　Questionnaire (TPQ), 16
　　BPD traits measured by, 21
Twin studies
　　of BPD, 36
　　of dissociative behaviors, 57
　　of personality traits, 29–31

Unshared variance,
   environmental influences,
   89–90

Verbal abuse, as psychological risk
   factor, 58–60

Youth suicide
   BPD, retrospective diagnosis
     of, 73–74
   cultural factors affecting, 75
   social disintegration and, 79
   substance abuse and, 74